INSPIRING PEOPLE

INSPIRING PEOPLE

Stories of Remarkable Recovery and Hope From The Gawler Foundation

Edited by Ian Gawler

THE GAWLER FOUNDATION

By the same Author:

You Can Conquer Cancer
Peace of Mind
Mind, Immunity and Health (Ed.)
New Cancer Perspectives (Ed.)
Mind, Immunity and Health II (Ed.)

Inspiring people: stories of remarkable recovery and hope
from The Gawler Foundation
Edited by Ian Gawler

Bibliography.
ISBN 0 9586461 0 4
1. Cancer – Treatment. 2. cancer – Patients – Biography.
I. Gawler, Ian, 1950–. II. Gawler Foundation.
362.1969940092

P.O. Box 77G, Yarra Junction, 3797, Australia
Tel: (059) 67 1730; Fax: (059) 67 1715

Typeset by Schuurman Computer Service
33 Don Road, Healesville Ph: (059) 62 2779
Typeset in Palatino 9.5/10.5

Inspiring People

These stories offer inspiration and very real hope. They are the true stories of people who have used the healing principles set out by Ian and Grace Gawler.

They were first told in the pages of The Gawler Foundation's newsletters. They are gathered together here and offered out of respect for those whose lives they recount, and in the hope that they will lead others towards the light of hope, positive action and a fulfilling life.

Most of the stories relate cases (often remarkable cases) of overcoming the physical symptoms of cancer. All of them relate remarkable journeys that involve transforming potential disaster and suffering into something quite fine. Some of the stories relate experiences of dying — dying well in a way that offers inspiration and hope for a good death — something we all must come to one day.

So these stories celebrate the efforts and lives of people affected by cancer — the patients themselves, the families, friends and therapists. Thanks are due to those who shared their lives in this way and may they be blessed by the benefits these stories offer to all who read them.

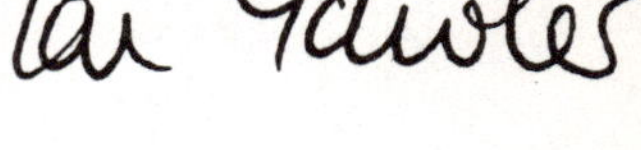

October 1995

Acknowledgements

The publisher would like to thank the contributors for sharing and writing their stories, Sue Dixon for the cover photo, Garth Davis and Village Roadshow for the cover design, Kate Thomas for proof reading, Robbie Schuurman for typesetting and the staff and volunteers at The Yarra Valley Living Centre for their help.

Contents

David Marriner

It is Monday, the day David spends at home, away from his busy commercial life as a property developer. Away from the hassles, excitements and challenges — like the Cumberland resort development at Lorne which is a current major project for him. David has just returned from 15 miles cycling and talks of being diagnosed as a cancer patient back in November 1983.

"It was devastating to be put in that position, especially being in a commercial position with major commitments and being the sole captain of your ship."

Surgery followed to remove the existing cancer and David felt fortunate "to have excellent assistance through that period from local and specialist medicos. But I was still devastated. The doctors said my cancer was a rarer than normal type and that they knew little about it. A week later I was fortunate to attend a Geelong seminar of Ian's and learned cancer was not a sentence. I gained hope which to that point had been lacking."

David then put in a great deal of effort with a commitment to change his diet. He travelled from his Colac home each week to attend the Melbourne cancer support group with Elaine his wife. "I went from French champagne and caviar to fruit juice and carrots! It was an effort but given the motivation it was easy. Being positive in my make up was a real plus and the change in diet and meditation played a big role in my overall wellbeing."

Elaine is a nursing sister. "It was an enormous commitment from her too, to change and learn in these new areas." David has seen others who have tried to change their eating habits but have been negative or envy their old ways. "You need an overall commitment from within the family unit. A number of factors help you at that critical point of being diagnosed. Not just one factor but a combination — wife, support group, meditation, diet and positive thinking.

"So many handle it as if it were a sentence. I was like this at first. It was hard, especially being married to a nurse who had nursed many dying cancer patients. Also, I felt as if the locals had kissed me goodbye, the business community too — it was a real problem. At the same time, I learnt of eight others locally who had cancer and had to live with the awareness that one by one they were dying. It was very trying. Elaine and I tried to pass on advice that had helped us so much.

We got to know the families and strong caring relationships developed. It was depressing to see others who did not make it.

"Coming to the support group and seeing others doing well reinforced our own real sense of hope. I took a great deal of comfort from thinking that only five to ten percent of my body was affected and that the rest was still working and that we could make it work better still."

"I see it as a real problem when people don't make a complete commitment. I have seen people who tried to make an effort and did improve their quality of life through improving their awareness and knowledge, but without that real commitment, they don't seem to get on top of it."

In mid 1984 David was forced back into work through financial pressure and dropped off the diet and meditation. As he travelled extensively, his exercise also fell away, while the stress levels rose.

"When I came home, Elaine said I wasn't looking too good and insisted I go for a blood test. The levels had gone up considerably and I was advised to start chemotherapy immediately. I got one hell of a fright. I blamed the results on how I had treated my body over the last two months and so, under medical supervision, delayed the treatment and got back onto my strict program. It took three to four tests before the levels began to come down but they were back to normal in six weeks. Although I did it without the chemotherapy, the medical people still find it hard to think that it was a result of this system."

"Now, 12 months later, I do travel a lot. We endeavour to be strict at home and I am prepared to relax a little when away. If we can't get the fresh orange juice we would have at home, then we are content to have other orange juice and be happy that at least it's not a beer. It is important to enjoy yourself. Now I am clear I have an occasional glass of wine whereas I didn't for 12 months.

"I am now back into a working routine and find my productivity is much greater than before. It has proved to me that my level of fitness and having my body and mind in balance helps greatly in my commercial life.

"There is real evidence that I have been able to advance commercially in the past nine months, undertake new issues and resolve them in more successful ways than before the illness.

"This is not something you should run away from once you are over the initial problems. You should keep it up and then you will be far better at what you used to do."

David, you demonstrate so well the value of making a full commitment, of making an effort both personally and as a family unit. Congratulations!

June 1986

Jean Fraser

Jean is a grandmother who has achieved something remarkable. She has become the second person we are aware of at The Gawler Foundation who has had a complete remission from pancreatic cancer — in the absence of any medical treatment.

It all began in January of 1985 when Jean, after a series of increasing difficulties, landed in hospital for a series of tests. A C.A.T. scan revealed a pancreas that had a very uneven surface — a mass of bumps. Cancer was confirmed by biopsy and Jean was devastated to learn that no treatment was to be recommended. She was advised to go home and "return when you turn yellow".

Jean remembers: "Of course I was determined that I did not want to die. After the doctor told us in the hospital, I recall packing up to go home. I said to Arnold my husband — "You get the car. I'll have a good cry and then meet you outside". As he left, I thought, "no I won't — I'll meditate instead — I am going to do something about this thing."

"My son Phillip lives in New York now and on hearing my news, he read everything he could and found out so much. Then a friend gave me The Gawler Foundation's address and it seems that here everything I wanted was being done.

"I attended the support group with Arnold and began to meditate for two hours each day. I changed my diet, cut out the salt, sugar and meat, and soon I felt better than I had for years.

"We decided to go for a holiday to New York and see the family there. It was a most relaxed and lovely time.

"When we returned, I thought it would be good to get a checkup and in October returned to my surgeon. He looked at my card and exclaimed, 'But that's amazing — that was all nine months ago.'

"He then felt my tummy," Jean continued, "and again appeared stunned. I asked him why and he said he could not feel any lumps and that he fully expected them to be there by now. When pressed he said he had expected me back in about three months from January as that was the normal progress.

"He then ordered X-rays and could not see any sign of the cancer although other pathologists were unsure. We also checked the original biopsy and a pathology expert confirmed the presence of cancer cells."

Jean then called in her brother, a consulting physician, who recommended a second opinion and another C.A.T. scan. The more detailed

C.A.T. scan showed that she does in fact now have a perfectly normal pancreas. She also has some puzzled doctors and a joyous family! Well done Jean!

December 1985

Bernice Grocke

Bernice Grocke has three daughters and five grandchildren. In 1980 she retired after 16 years of running a gift shop and began doing voluntary work for Rubella children.

In October 1980 Bernice found that a mole on her leg was in fact a melanoma. 'My heavens,' I thought, 'it happens to others but not to me.' I wasn't really angry — but I had cancer.

Treatment was the surgical removal of the lump with a 6" x 4" resection and a skin graft to replace it.

"I was told there were three types of melanoma: one was harmless, one needed to be carefully watched, and the other was fatal. Mine was the second type. I was told it was all taken but it may come back and to watch it."

Regular check-ups followed and in the middle of 1983 two lumps appeared in the groin. Having been led to expect it, Bernice managed the second surgery all right but in 1984 began to feel 'horribly ill.'

A check-up revealed nothing obvious and she was advised to return in three months. She went earlier. A C.A.T. scan revealed melanoma secondaries in both lungs.

"I was told that nobody could help me and was sent for a second opinion. Again I was told that there was no treatment. The specialist did say, 'Of course there is Ainslie Meares and Ian Gawler, but really nobody can help.'

"So I rang Ian and in September 1984 joined the group with my husband Wain. With his help, I really got stuck into it very earnestly. I thought, 'if there is a chance of living, I want to.' I kept telling myself how much I was needed. My husband and children need me and my grandchildren will need me.

"I stuck rigidly to the daily program, finding the diet easy. The meditation was a problem at first; my mind kept wandering around others in the group and things to do with cancer.

"The group was very helpful, there was a great atmosphere and the meditation was better there. At home my mind kept wandering.

"Then Wain and I went for a weekend away and we went into a dear little historic church at Port Fairy. On a wall was a plaque which caught my eye: *'Be still and know that I am God'*. It seemed just right for me, being a Christian used to prayer.

"So I began to meditate by relaxing first then starting with this and saying it over and over. I also sang it to myself like a little mantra, until I felt absolutely still.

"Knowing so many friends were praying for me was a wonderful help also. One day I thought, why not let the meditation take the form of prayer. So I began to pray for everyone in the group by name and this led me into a very deep meditation. Then I prayed for everyone worldwide with cancer and then for myself, especially the painful parts — my back especially was very painful.

"This all led me into a great stillness.

"I had days when I was very down, however the support of the family was excellent. Having Wain at the groups was wonderful because he knew what I was doing.

"One night, if it were not for Wain, I would have given it in. He said, 'What are you?' I just turned away. 'Come on,' he said, 'You are a positive person now.' Repeating the affirmation for me triggered a response and I picked up.

"After a while, I felt that if I was dying I didn't feel too bad. My pain was down and after six months my surgeon said I was looking remarkably well. 'I feel it,' I replied. So I had a scan in February 1985 and it showed my left lung clear and the right one improved!

"In another six months I was feeling better and better and everyone was noticing it. In September 1985, another scan showed both lungs clear — 'perfectly normal,' the specialist said.

"When the left lung had been cleared, I crowed to the world. I told everyone. Now, this was so precious, so special, I wanted to keep it to myself. I shared it with the family, of course, but I was filled with a joy so exquisite that I just wanted to hug it to myself for a while before telling everyone.

One specialist said he could not understand it, whereas the other specialist and my G.P. are very enthusiastic and have asked me to speak to other patients to help them.

"I now feel and look so well, that every day I give thanks to God and I continue to pray for others."

June 1986

Rhonda Preston

"Dear Ian —

This is a thank you letter — a success story. Please allow me to briefly fill you in.

In September 1983 I had a mastectomy for breast cancer. The surgery was followed by a five week course of ray treatment. In August 1985 early liver secondaries were picked up in a routine liver scan and ultra-sound. I was devastated — being a trained nurse I fully understood the implications of the diagnosis. I was also angered that this should happen to me — particularly as I'd always taken responsibility for my health. My doctors felt that the cancer may be hormonal sensitive and suggested an oophorectomy (I'm 44) which was carried out a few days later.

Soon after this surgery, I was fortunate enough to hear of your weekend seminar at the A.N.U. here in Canberra and I went along, in hindsight the best thing I could ever have done. You were a great inspiration to me — I came away full of courage and thinking more positively than I had for years, determined to follow your regime.

I had read Ainslie Meares *Relief Without Drugs* some years previously and had learned some relaxation techniques, but now started meditating. After a few false starts it didn't take me long to begin to have some success, although I had good and bad days and only now feel able to slide into a state of meditation with relative ease. I meditated for about two hours a day — preceding the sessions with devotional reading and prayer. (Being a bit of a back-slider in the past, prayer was not always easy — I felt such a fraud daring to ask for help only when I was in trouble.) I visualised my body internally and turned my mind inwardly upon my cancer. I exhorted my body defences to get cracking and reject this intruder. When driving alone in the car I talked non-stop to myself. I forbade the cancer to get any bigger — imagined it starving through lack of oestrogen.

I embraced the diet fully. This was the least difficult thing for me to do. Being more or less a vegetarian for several years I did not suffer the trauma of giving up Sunday roast etc. Fortunately I've never had a sweet-tooth. But tea and coffee were hard at first!

I persevered and persevered and although I had days when I was in the pits I kept fairly well, helped by the support of family (husband, daughter 19 and son 17) and friends. I went back to work (I work in a school for handicapped children) and although I woke each morning with a realisation of dread, I had inner resources (God given) to overcome this and meditation to rely on. What a tool meditation is! It brought me to inner peace, comfort and courage. I was determined not to be too afraid of dying to enjoy the living.

Being a nurse was limiting to me — I didn't really believe a cure possible, but I believed and knew that with these new tools I now possessed I would live as long as possible with maximum quality.

In November 1985 my doctor ordered another liver scan to see if the cancer was influenced by oophorectomy and to check on its size.

I couldn't believe it — no one else could — but there was no evidence of a progressive carcinoma, just some "scarring" on the site of the tumour. In April this year a further scan was done which was totally clear — even the scarring could not be detected.

You can imagine how thankful I feel. My doctors are saying very little about the whole thing apart from the fact that they feel the oophorectomy was the treatment which 'seems to have done the trick.' I agree up to a point, but when I mention meditation and diet they are very polite and listen and are even a bit patronising. I *know* they are shortchanging the value of meditation, positive thinking etc. and I feel so frustrated at these attitudes. However I will continue to quietly uphold them in the hope that someone else can be helped. One doctor even muttered that perhaps I never had secondaries — he was the same medico who said of the original diagnosis (when I, in a state of denial, queried it) that there couldn't possibly be a mistake.

I will always continue to meditate and I wouldn't think of eating any other way. I feel so well, so fit and life is better than ever. For the first time I've got my life together spiritually (belief in a higher being — in my case God), mentally (meditation and positive attitudes) and physically (diet etc.) and I feel jus great. Thank you Ian.

Yours most sincerely,

Rhonda Preston

P.S. I apologise for this "brief" letter turning out to be so long."

June 1986

Jim Malliaros

Jim was diagnosed on August 9th, 1984 as having terminal cancer of the prostate gland. It had spread to his spine, pelvis and the back of the ribs. Jim's future was bleak and it affected him badly. In his own words:

"Like most people who have been told that they face a situation similar to mine the idea of cancer inevitably meant death. Death was to me a subject I associated with other people; the old, the sick or the lonely, and like most people I took it for granted. However when I was told that death was a real possibility in the very near future my initial shock was great — my health in the past had never been of any real concern.

"The next few weeks were spent with each day meaning that I was closer to death than the day before. My whole lifestyle seemed to be one of 'no future'; I felt as if I had nothing to live for and sometimes I felt as though I might as well die now to stop all the suffering of the days ahead.

"Because of their situation with forthcoming exams, my wife and I decided against telling our two teenage children; however they too soon discovered the change in my way of life and we knew the news should be broken soon. My wife tried very hard to provide the love and attention to myself (to whom the doctors had given no hope) but the word 'cancer' was taboo and we tried to ignore it.

"One day while at the newsagency (about three months after my diagnosis) I noticed a book near the newspaper I was going to buy called *You Can Conquer Cancer.* I decided to buy it and after reading only the first few pages my initial thoughts centred around the idea of 'If he can do it, then so can I'. Through the book and all that it had to offer, I became aware of The Australian Cancer Patients Foundation and so I quickly enrolled as a member and joined a particular group.

"What I learned at the Centre was:

- Hope: I began to think of the future, not just sickness and death.
- Understanding: I talked with people in the same position.
- Encouragement: I met people who had beaten cancer.
- Positive thinking: and the powers of the mind.
- Meditation: which helps my healing process.

- Diet: which promotes health of the body.

and most importantly:

- Happiness: (as a result of all the above): which had not been a part of my life for quite a while.

This ability to control and cope with stress and illness through meditation, diet and positive thinking has given me a new identity and now even my family are eating the type of food that I eat and are meditating with me. They say that they too have discovered more about life and themselves as a result of their and my 'improved lifestyle'."

Jim has become keen to help others now he is feeling so much better. Greek born, Jim has visited several other Greek cancer patients and has been able to overcome the language barrier that sometimes exists for these people. Now Jim's ever-ready wit is helping others to laugh and look on the bright side, and he is an inspiration to many.

Jim has the wonderful gift of being able to share his positive experiences with others.

October 1985

August 1986 — An Update

Jim has some insights to add now:

Jim says that "initially I had a big problem in attending Ian's talks. On the one hand I knew that I had the best doctors and they were saying there was no hope for me. Yet here it all seemed so simple. When I started the course I found the first three or four lessons unconvincing and because of this I did not believe Ian's ideas and methods would help me to cure my cancer. However, after a few more lessons, I slowly started to become convinced. By this stage, all the people in the group started talking freely to each other about their problems which helped enormously in our friendship and made all of us extremely happy."

During 1985 Jim kept coming to The Gawler Foundation, "because I found I was becoming a different person, a better person from when I started, and I was living a happier life than before. I went again to completely clarify all I was learning and found the extra sessions extremely beneficial. Now any time that I feel that I am losing the importance of these ideas I quickly go back to The Gawler Foundation to reinforce them."

During 1985 Jim continued to look better and better. Urged to go for more tests and scans, Jim refused. Jim kept in touch with his doctors but as for detailed tests, he said: "I don't want to know", his eyes closed and arms up in characteristic Greek fashion! "I feel great. If the cancer is still there or worse, I don't want to know, I can't do any more and it's O.K. If the cancer has gone, I still don't want to change anything. I'm enjoying life. I could die tomorrow but I expect to live a long time again now."

Finally in April 1986, Jim relented and had full tests conducted. "I was very surprised and quite elated to find that there was no trace of it anywhere in my body." A full remission when no medical treatment was available!

Jim continues to nurture his good health, maintaining his diet, meditation and positivity. He also acts as an inspiration to many via the voluntary contact group and often spends hours with other people and their families (especially Greeks) just starting on the road he has walked. It is wonderful to see him giving so much of his experience to others.

June 1992 — A Tribute to a Friend

Many members and friends of The Gawler Foundation will have been saddened by the news of Jim's death. While Jim's life was a miracle to celebrate, the fact that he is no longer walking amongst us, spreading his hope and good humour, is really saddening.

Jim was one of those exceptional beings who, having experienced a remarkable, medically unexpected recovery, marvelled at what happened for him and wanted to share the good news. He gave so much of himself in voluntary service, visiting those recently diagnosed in their homes or hospital, often calling on others in advanced illness. Always the same message: there is hope, you can help yourself, your family and friends can make a difference, life is worth living, make the effort, it will be repaid in full.

My guess is that some will be unsettled by Jim's death. He had come to be another prominent symbol of what is possible. That cancer can be overcome not only in living with it and being the better for the experience of it, but in actually recovering physically.

I know that Jim was concerned about this impact of his declining health and his death approaching. It was good to have been able to talk with him again a few days before he did die and remind him of his triumph. He survived some seven years longer than expected. He brought inspiration, hope and real health and peace to literally hundreds, perhaps thousands of others in real need. I told him how I had come to love him and how many others held him in their love.

Jim's was a great life, made greater by his response to the huge challenge presented by cancer and all he subsequently helped. Please pray for him and hold him dear in your heart during meditation. And offer your support to his wife Angela and the boys.

For those of us fortunate enough to know this man, Jim Malliaros' life was a miracle.

Ian Gawler

The Seven Day Live-in Program
A Patient's Perspective

By Gary Sutherland — April 1986

The April seven-day live-in program was held at Jumbunna Lodge, overlooking the beautiful Yarra Valley, near Yarra Junction.

The week brought together a group of people (cancer patients and support people) from all over Australia and even as far away as New Zealand. Perhaps it was a reflection of my own feelings going into the week, but I met a group of people who at first sight seemed dispirited and whose eyes were dulled with a sense of despair.

In an atmosphere that nurtured love, sharing, caring and a joy for living, people responded openly, honestly, at times emotionally. I will be forever thankful for the opportunity to be a part of this week. Ian, Grace and David shared a wealth of life experiences and knowledge that were an inspiration to all who were there.

Ian led sessions dealing with:

- Meditation — one of life's truly simple pleasures;
- Positive thinking — "If you think you can or you think you cannot, you're right" — quote by Henry Ford;
- Creative thinking — using mental images and affirmations to change life goals and how we perceive ourselves;
- Pain — "does it really have to hurt?";
- Death and dying — a realistic, reassuring look into the "too hard basket".

Ian facilitated the skills needed for small group discussions that for me, were intense, revealing, yet free of intrusion beyond people's capacity to give. The overwhelming response of people was a sense of privilege to be involved.

What better tonic can there be than the double-edged sword of wisdom and wit. To Ian, Chris and Denis, I thank you. For me, "wind" will henceforth be associated with the state of my digestion rather than the weather. A support person will always be to me a martyr with a sense of humour.

Grace shared with us her principles of good eating: adopting positive attitudes, choosing appropriate food, good ways to prepare food. She contributed a degree of vitality, energy, empathy and support that would have tumour cells surrendering to the nearest lymphocyte. Grace is a shining example of a happy, well adjusted martyr.

Both the venue and the program promoted the idea of exercise being important to physical and mental well-being. As an active person I would have liked more time to be physically active. David provided the stimulus and leadership for early morning exercises. Through David's guidance with breathing exercises I re-introduced my lungs to oxygen and so began the process of making friends with my body again.

For me, this week neither promised nor gave out cures for cancer. It did however provide the rational basis for developing a lifestyle that is in harmony (physically, emotionally, mentally and spiritually) with my world, my family and friends.

Clearly, there seems little doubt that we all must die. How we wish to live is the choice and challenge that we face. My life has reached a crisis point that has real danger associated with it. It wasn't until this week that I realized the opportunity for healing that went with it. The choice is obvious, but not easy, but there is a choice and, for me, hope. The fear associated with the danger I face is real, but now controllable, so that it mobilizes the body's natural defences. It is well documented what people are capable of when their life is in danger and they choose to fight. This week has shown clearly for me that my fight is with cancer, not death. This is a fight I can and will win. To Ian and Grace and the A.C.P.F., thank you hardly seems enough, but written in words, that is how it comes out.

June 1986

Bill Lees

This delightful story comes directly as told by Bill. As Bill explains, he did it upon request in hospital. He was asked to "get out of bed and tell the Gawler story to six ladies in bed recovering from chemo. It is a bit rough, but an honest assessment. I only did it to help others in need and trust it will.

"My name is Edwin (Bill) Lees, and I am now well into my 79th year and reside at Cowes, Phillip Island, with my wife Marjorie, who played a large part in my fight to remove cancer completely from my body.

"During a period when I was an in-patient I mentioned that I had been successful in removing cancer from my body, over a progressive period, from late 1988 to remission in 1990. Early February 1991 I received a bone scan report. No mestatic disease evident.

"I was asked, would I tell my story on tape so that it could be used to demonstrate to people with cancer that there was an option available to them that had a proven success rate, wherein you use the resources of your body to destroy the cancer.

"My story could ramble on in detail for a long time so I will endeavour to keep it as brief as possible and trust that the important facets will assist others in their fight against cancer. It should, however, be kept in mind that throughout my fight I had a total commitment to the Gawler program of teaching and training methods over a period of two years, until I got my cancer into remission. Even now, we observe all the main facets of the program, meditation, a sensible but broader diet, exercise, avoiding stress of any kind and maintaining peace of mind and body.

"Meditation is the important key and stress is the enemy.

"During late 1985 I had a prostate operation and was advised after that there was no cancer evident, a grey area, yes, but pathology cleared it as non-malignant, as I was informed by my oncologist.

"In March 1988 I again had a prostate problem and on investigation by the same oncologist he advised that I had a malignant cancer and that it was nasty, no further explanation, however. I was advised to have an orchiectomy operation (removal of my testicles). This would stop the production of testosterone, which was a very good food for cancer. In due course I had this operation and I believe it was one of the best decisions I made as it did assist in the overall success of the complete removal of cancer from my body.

"As I was booked to go overseas at this time, it was agreed that I delay the operation and take special medication that would protect against any spread of the cancer. I had a bone scan before departure to make sure that I had no secondary bone cancer and as the result was no secondary bone cancer I went merrily on my way with friends. However, I took ill two months into the trip and on return I had another bone scan, only to find that I had extensive secondary bone cancer in the rib cage and pelvic area.

"The urologist passed me over to an oncologist who insisted that I immediately have the ophorectomy operation and declared my condition as terminal with an expectancy of six to 12 months.

"At the age of 78 I decided not to have chemotherapy and went looking for a Pritikin 1980 diet book to indulge in a good diet. I came across Ian Gawler's book *You Can Conquer Cancer* with great emphasis on the *you;* not I can cure your cancer. This book was the key to the health I enjoy today at close to 80 years and enabled me to remove cancer completely from my body.

"To achieve this result you must be both dedicated and positive to the teachings and training.

"A brief summary of Ian & Graces' story is in the front of his book *You Can Conquer Cancer* and believe me they overcame an impossible cancer, went on to get married, have a family and set up a training to give people with cancer the benefit of all the experiences that enabled them to kill their cancer.

"I got in touch with the Gawler office at Yarra Junction and entered one of their early live-in (10 days) training programs on 11 November 1988. I can state here and now that it was the turning point of my life. Not only did I succeed in removing cancer from my body, I also changed my life-style for a much happier and healthier and relaxed way of life and this reflected onto my family and many friends, through their adoption of the many excellent procedures.

"I could not possibly explain in full detail the live-in program. It is intensive in every respect and on-going for the full 10 days, covering gentle exercises, meditation and training, diet and all about how to live your life from there on. It is truly an inspiration and learning experience not to be missed.

"Basically — meditation to generate peace of mind (calm both mind and body), diet and exercise to build up the immune system (with the aid of supplements) and exercise to keep the body fit and relaxed etc. The training also includes how you should view and live your life from there on and it is all good.

"My wife and I quickly settled down to living the Gawler way and quickly conquered the new and enjoyable way of life.

My progress was rapid — peace of mind and a good diet does that, plus the confidence in your mind that you are conquering your cancer.

"I do sincerely trust this story will be of some help to those people fighting cancer or desiring to avoid it.

"My only advice is to act quickly and positively in your fight to destroy your cancer. Do not delay. The decision is yours."

The Quality of Life (Self-Help for Cancer Patients)

An article from Colleen O'Connell who attended the April seven-day program — courtesy of the Tallangatta Herald, 25th June, 1986:

"In April this year I was fortunate enough to have the opportunity to attend a seven day live-in program conducted by the Australian Cancer Patients Foundation. I would like to share this very worthwhile experience with others.

Although The Foundation's main concern is self-help techniques for cancer patients, it also organises "healthy living" programs with no emphasis on cancer as such. The clinic I attended was for cancer patients and their main support person. Approximately 42 people were in attendance and ages ranged from mid-twenties to sixty plus.

During our seven day retreat we were treated to lectures on good food awareness and preparation, creative thinking, pain control, relaxation, meditation and philosophy on death and dying. Our diet for the week was strictly vegetarian with significance placed on raw food. Sugar, salt, meat, chicken, fish, coffee, tea (except herbal teas), artificial additives, and highly refined foods were nowhere in sight. Of course smoking was not even a consideration.

The transformation in the members of the group as the week progressed was nothing short of amazing. Some had arrived a little wary and unsure whilst others had a very enthusiastic and open minded approach. Others had a look of helplessness, despairing, confusion and a few even appeared to have lost the will to live. However, the whole group became happy, enlightened, positive people. We all departed as loving, caring friends who had a definite path to follow in a very meaningful and purposeful manner.

The sessions were conducted by Ian Gawler, Director of The Foundation, his wife Grace and another Foundation member, David MacRae. Ian was a terminally ill cancer patient over 10 years ago and at one stage was given two weeks to live. He is living proof of self-help principles as he was declared completely clear of cancer in July 1978. He also has four children, eight years and under, and leads a very active and satisfying life.

Despite the phrase "cancer is a word and not a sentence", few people appear to believe it. One of Ian's positive thinking, self-help philosophies is a quote by Henry Ford, "If you think you can or you think you cannot, you're right." Another favourite was "The only thing you can't do is not die (eventually). You can do what you strive to do, just have a positive attitude and believe totally in what you are doing."

I would like to recommend The Foundation to not only cancer patients and their families, but everyone in general. Ian Gawler's book *You Can Conquer Cancer* details The Foundation's program and is very worthwhile reading. It is relevant to mention that a change in life-style can help with any emotional or physical disability and is not exclusive for cancer patients. While there is life there is hope and the quality of life is important.

To sum up my once-in-a-lifetime experience, I found it very rewarding and enlightening. I am pleased to say that this experience has flowed onto my personal relationships, and I can detect a move towards a more harmonious family life.

Needless to say, the chemical free vegies have been lovingly planted and antibiotic free chickens are next in the melting pot! (The chook pen is under construction). I just have to deter my husband from spraying nearby paddocks — now that will take a lot of positive manoeuvring!"

August 1986

Barbara Harkness
From the Re-creation Program

In November 1991 Barbara attended a six-day residential program at the Yarra Valley Living Centre. Earlier in the year she wrote an account of what was happening in her life before she attended the residential and what then happened. It provides great inspiration and incentive for us all. No matter how stuck we may feel it is always possible to find a way forward through the gentle focus of meditation and the power of sharing in a loving and safe environment.

A Lesson in Subjective Pain

Background: 5th November 1991

"My life to this point was burdened by years of unresolved grief stemming from a childhood which had been both traumatic and socially isolated. Events of deepest scarring included psychological, physical and emotional abuse by an overly aggressive father and the sudden death of an uncle which coincided with the dislocation of migrating to Australia. Adolescence culminated in a nervous breakdown and attempted suicide at age 16.

"Twenty-one years later I continued to suffer from resultant depression which was exacerbated by an incident at the Flinders Medical Centre in November 1990. The difficult insertion and mis-management of an intravenous drip line in my right wrist (to facilitate the administration of antibiotic therapy) led to subsequent thrombophlebitis. This was particularly distressing as I was assured on admission (by doctors) that there was no possibility of any complications to this procedure. I was misinformed. My condition was further compounded emotionally by the attitude of doctors and nursing staff (both at the hospital and during further treatment) who all appeared to support the 'compliance' model of health care which treats the illness and ignores the patient.

"Dequervain's tenosynovitis and an entrapment of the superficial branch of the radial nerve were diagnosed some months later. I had also developed a panic reaction to hospitals and a deep mistrust of the medical profession. An orthopaedic surgeon in whom I held some confidence operated in July 1991 bringing some relief of the symptoms but

Ruth Croft-Firman

Ruth Firman, from Perth, is one of those wonderful people who did it. She recovered from cancer. Since then she has continued to help many other new patients both individually and in groups. Hers is a truly inspiring story.

"It is now twenty years since a 'Pap' smear indicated endometrial cancer of my womb just early enough for surgery to save my life. Cancer in first the left then the right lung followed — fortunately with early enough chest X-rays for a lobectomy of each lung. In 1985 metastasies in the right lung gave me a "Sorry, nothing more can be done" verdict, but through the Cancer Support Association I heard a doctor who was a guest speaker suggest intensive meditation had helped some of his patients.

I went to him and then meditated, as he asked, for three hours a day in half-hour sessions using the audio taped peaceful imagery he provided. I took a small portable recorder everywhere and sat in the oddest places to ensure I didn't miss a session, even sitting in public toilets to gain privacy after a man in the street looked into my car and panicked thinking my slack facial muscles meant I was dead!

Later, with the doctor's approval, I wrote my own words for another audio tape with specific, positive health statements aimed at guiding my immune system. In the audio tape I also stated, "I am completely at peace, happy and contented", which was a direct contradiction of my feelings when I began using it. I was surprised when about a month later I realised I felt at peace and happy, despite no outward changes in my life situation.

I was amazed when only three months of this intensive three-hour-a-day meditation resulted in my first clear X-ray. Since then all my six-monthly chest X-rays have stayed clear of cancer and my chest physician said recently that annual visits are now enough. I rewarded him with a gift of one of my large water colours! Fortunately he liked it.

Back in 1985, once my X-rays were clear, I surprised my family when I booked in to see Dr Ainslie Meares in Melbourne. They accepted the idea, but thought it strange for me to want to do this now my lungs were clear. But I considered it important to have the best help available to ensure I maintained my return to good health.

I had about two weeks with Dr Meare's *natural* meditation method. But when I heard of Ian Gawler's first seminar, I broke into my time with Dr Meares to go to it. I found Ian's 1985 seminar wonderful, especially as I recognised how much of his theoretical base had quite a lot in common with a TAFE further education course I had written on creativity. But Ian had brilliantly transferred these theories to aim at establishing good health and well-being.

I realised my audio taped messaged had quite a lot of basic similarity to Ian's theory and I think they were possibly very powerful when I was listening to them in my own voice during deeply relaxed intensive meditation. Especially as the life statements were of my own choosing.

Although I began with audio tapes, I now mostly use Dr Ainslie Meare's *natural* method, except when I want to change some of my attitudes or bring about major changes in my life. I find these happen very naturally. But, I always use a 'trigger phrase' to cue my mind into deep relaxation. Once I say to myself, "I am relaxing easily ... quickly ... and deeply', this repeated 'trigger phrase' takes me immediately into a relaxed state to begin a session. In fact, it now makes the conscious relaxing of each muscle automatic, as it eases my mind quickly into relaxation.

Trevor Steele

Trevor Steele received a rather unusual fortieth birthday present — a diagnosis of widespread non-Hodgkins lymphoma.

Having worked for twenty years in youth and community welfare, Trevor had been suffering extreme tiredness since September 1985. Repeated blood tests had all showed negative; the advice was to eat good food and rest.

Trevor agonized over what was happening to him. Finally his weight loss became acute and lumps appeared around his neck. On his 40th birthday the biopsy was performed. Then a seven day wait. The process of being ushered into the doctor's rooms by a nurse, being checked by another to see he was seated, the doctor coming in, drawing his chair up close. By then it was hardly a surprise — widespread cancer, being booked into a specialist cancer hospital, no treatment except chemotherapy possible, fear and apprehension. What does it all mean? Is the hospital for treatment or somewhere to go to die? The message was "you are booked in, they are very good, they will tell you what will happen." The conclusion could only be that the prognosis was poor.

Trevor rang relatives and friends to break the news. Most were stunned, shocked. Then he rang a health resort manager. "I told him I had cancer. 'Wow', he said, 'isn't that great!'(It was my turn to drop the phone!) He said that there were all sorts of opportunities to find out what life is all about and you have chosen a real good one.'

"Something clicked with the word 'choice'. I had not read any of Ian Gawler's or John Harrison's stuff, but I figured if I could choose to give myself the disease I could give it away. It was a new idea, but it had a great impact. He also said, 'You are in for the greatest adventure of your life.' My reaction was, 'Some adventure, I may be dead next week.' But the adventure thing came up again. Just before I left for the hospital, I went to the local doctor. She said, 'Don't get sucked into the tunnel down there, it's your life, you are in charge.' I went out feeling a bit angry, thinking that's alright for her, she knows cancer; but this is happening to me and it's pretty frightening. I went into a bookshop and the first book that hit me was on the factual aspects of cancer. I got to know what this thing called lymphoma was. It said chemotherapy gave a 0–20% chance of survival after five years. It was enough ammunition to ask intelligent questions when I got to the hospital.

"In fact, it all seemed to happen in that week before hospital. A series of what appeared at first to be unrelated circumstances led to it all coming together.

"The night before leaving for hospital I went to visit my manager from work. I was expressing my fears and then he gave me the most incredible feeling of optimism and confidence. He helped me to see that there was a lot I wanted to live for.

"The next day, I bounced up to the counter at the hospital and said, 'Hi! I am here to learn as much about cancer as I can.' They said, 'Are you sure you are in the right place?'

"I had brought a walkman cassette player to begin playing relaxing music. I also took it into my consultations and asked to record them all. This had the effect of letting the doctors know that I was going to seriously consider all they said. I imagined that I would be overwhelmed with facts and would need to refer to the tape. In fact, I never have, but it did let my attitude be known.

"Looking at the other patients, they were so sick and unhappy, I really felt that I was in the wrong place. However, C.A.T. scans confirmed secondary spread in my lymph nodes of stomach, spleen and groin. The advice was for chemotherapy and that I should start in a week's time. I said I wanted time to consider it and see if I could do it my way. So they sent me to the social worker. It seems her job was to get me to do what the doctors said and I was quite shocked by that.

"By the time I went back for another visit, I had investigated diets. I told the social worker I was using vitamin supplements and watching my diet. With the help of a G.P. I was following a well monitored program aimed at stimulating my immune system. She advised I see the hospital dietitian. I thought that was a bit of a laugh as they had just given me lunch! White bread sandwiches with sausage and plastic cheese plus canned soup.

"I felt that a lot of her concerns revolved around me being a single male living on my own and her doubts that I could prepare a balanced diet. I did talk with the dietitian and he felt that what I was doing was OK without acknowledging that diet could assist recovery.

"The doctors continued to push me to have chemotherapy. They said it was my only chance. I said thanks, but I want to try it my way first. I had read a little now and chemotherapy did not feel right for me. It did not make sense to have it depleting my immune system when I wanted to built it up. I began looking at all ways possible to stimulate my immune system."

Diet was to become a major focus for Trevor's healing efforts. It was the tangible thing he did while he continued working on the inside. It was something that his parents related to directly also. So when he showed an interest in wheatgrass, his mother took it on as a labour of love to keep him in supplies of the freshly grown sprouted wheat. It was a good way for her to become involved and show her support.

Trevor's actual work situation was full of challenges also.

In December of 1985 he had resigned his social work job. From March 1986, Trevor began working at Hepburn Springs' new complex as a massseur. "This added to my fears of hopelessness, helplessness. I had switched from employee to self-employed — in a new field where there was no idea of the projections.

"For the next three months I was too weak to work. Some days I could avoid the worries, but the bills kept rolling in and some days were down. Then I got sickness benefit which helped.

Next I went to the residential program in July 1986. This got me more on the right track with diet and I started meditation which was very powerful. I also came away with very clear affirmations — 'I am a well person now.' That was how I felt. I came away from it with a deep inner knowing that I was well. There was something wrong with being on a sickness benefit and feeling like that, so I stopped the benefit and recommenced work.

"I realized that there are two types of people: happy ones and unhappy ones. If you put an unhappy person into a good situation it will not take long before that person will find something to complain about. Likewise a happy person can find something to be grateful and happy about in any situation. I realized I could choose to be happy and this became an affirmation. If you have cancer, why be unhappy as well? I chose to be happy.

"Things seemed to come alive. Sunrises seemed more beautiful and warmer, flowers seemed brighter and smelt sweeter, everything had more impact on me. This kept reinforcing the feeling that I could maintain the happy feeling, and it has worked.

"I had several people early in the piece ask me if I was married or had a family, and when I said no they said, 'That's lucky' or 'That's good'. The inference was rather staggering. It was at a time when I would really have liked someone to share the journey with. I felt horribly alone. However, I can realize now what a strength that gave me. The illness was something only I could deal with.

"I sent a letter to all my friends sharing how positive I was feeling. It was to try and show them that I was coping well. Some I never heard from again! Either they could not handle it or they thought that I was coping so well I needed no help. That was not what I meant at all! I wanted some attention! As it happened, I recovered pretty quickly. After a couple of months being back at work and looking well, everyone expected me to be well and treated me as such.

"Recently I got locked into long work hours again. Feeling exhausted and having aches in my stomach and legs, I went back to hospital for the first tests and C.A.T. scans in 12 months. Thinking there would be nothing there, I felt, that's no good, how can I justify a holiday if I am well. Suddenly it really struck me that this illness gave me an excuse to do some of the things I wanted to.

"What showed up in the scan was exactly the same as the original scans two years ago. I have had no conventional treatments at all. I was a bit disappointed. The doctors said there was no sign of progression and so they recommended no treatment. It was quite a step down for them after having said the chemo was my only hope two years ago. At that time it was recorded that I had stubbornly refused treatment and instead taken up 'expensive alternative treatment.' It seems my doctors at that time felt that was the best way to describe eating good food and taking vitamins and minerals and vitamin C injections. They also said that while it was likely what I was intending to do would cause no harm, there was no way meditation could help my outcome. I went for a second opinion to another specialist who said there was no way it could not. I preferred his more positive approach!

"When I had been for a check up after about 12 months, I had seen a new doctor at the hospital. He had said that he liked to evaluate results and if I was so well after no treatment then whatever I was doing was working very well.

"As time goes on, new insights keep coming. Understanding the cause of the disease was greatly helped by attending a seminar with Dr. John Harrison, author of *Love Your Disease*. John spoke of the reasons for getting a disease and it hit me again why I still needed it. I still had not got all the attention I needed after I recovered so quickly. However, I realized that now I do not need an excuse. Now I know I don't need to be sick to justify being kind to myself. I can take time out for me because I need it and I don't need any other reason.

"Over the last two years I have noticed that when I have fears things don't go well. When I let them go, life begins to flow and the law of synchronicity operates — things just seem to happen at the right time.

"With cancer, the realization that I could die led me to start living and to make the most of every moment of every day.

"At the moment, I know I can give the cancer away if I want to. I feel that if I had a scan now it would be clear as I no longer need the illness.

"As I put into practice all I have learnt through having had cancer, I feel the sky is the limit in my life now."

October 1988

The Wild Rover
Reflections on the 7-day Program

... One of the most powerful experiences of my life — Trevor Steele

On the last day of the July 7-day program, Trevor delighted all attending with his rendition of "The Wild Rover" — sung with a definite lilt! Due to popular demand, here is the edited version:

I've been a wild rover for many a year
But I've never struck anythin' like I've struck 'ere ...
At a Centre out 'ere midst the rolling green hills
They do nothin' but focus on all of yer ills.

CHORUS:
An' it's no, no never
Never anywhere else
Never ever before 'ave I seen
A place so obsessed with yer 'ealth.

If a bloke wants a smoke or a wee 'armless drink
There's people out 'ere makes 'im first stop and think
Think of 'is lungs and think of 'is 'eart,
They say ya gotta stop now and make a fresh start.

They started the rot when — just like back in school
They made us draw pictures — I felt such a fool!
Their trick was to get me to let it all out
Then they'd somehow interpret what me life's all about.

We did breathin' and chantin' of every kind ...
Relaxin' the body and stillin' the mind.
But 'tho I felt like a rag doll ... me head was still buzzin'
With thoughts floodin' through at fourteen to the dozen.

Images and visions and bright healing lights
We did it ad nauseum from mornin' till night
It annoyed me to do it at Ian's every whim —
I mean, the lotus position's dead easy for 'im!

And I found affirmations a bit 'ard to take
Despite what I said, me mind knew it was false
It's really much more than a bloke can endure
'Cos I only came 'ere for some magical cure.

The remedy prescribed by their "Dr. MacRae"
Was a "meditation cocktail" — taken four times a day.
But we have no doubt, as we sift through all this chaff
The best medicine of all is a bloody good laugh!

Grace's quite amazing ... she's real living proof
Of the value in dryin' yer grapes on the roof.
But I asked her one question I'm sorry she answer'd —
No bloke likes to 'ear that 'is nuts 'ave gone rancid!

Now the group of us 'ere — we're not such a bad lot
But we've all now damn near 'ad enough of this rot;
One more day in this place and we'd surely revolt ...
I'd give me right arm for a spoonful of salt.

So if yer riddled with cancer and you've lost all yer drive
And ya really see no point in stayin' alive
Don't go to the Gawlers, 'cos no matter 'ow 'ard ya try
They'll 'ave ya stay 'ealthy
Till the day that ya die!

August 1986

Sylvia Moss

Sylvia's story highlights the needs to manage stress and the benefits that come with doing just that.

The first physical sign that something was wrong for Sylvia came back in 1981 when she began developing a severe stitch in her side while playing tennis. Sylvia had never been really sick in her life up to now, but she was aware that things were not right in her life. There were problems at home and she just could not talk it through with her husband. He was thinking of leaving her.

"I felt worried and tensed up inside. There was a lot of tension and stress and everything was being just bottled up inside. The pain in my side got worse but I tried to ignore it. Then I developed diarrhoea but the doctor just thought I had a gastro virus. Only when I started vomiting did I have X-rays and a tumour in my bowel was discovered."

Sylvia was fortunate. The tumour was still small and could be removed easily and completely by surgery. Her husband stayed on with the family and things went well until late 1984. Her husband left.

"At that time I am sure I could easily have gone under. Looking back, I was sure that stress had helped bring the cancer on in the first place, and now I was very distressed — devastated.

"I had been very dependent upon my husband — I could not believe that he would not come back. I had never been independent.

"I was really low when my sister, who was worried that I would get sick again, organized me to come to the support group.

"At first it was hard, but the meditation was fantastic for me. Perhaps more importantly, I realized that I still did have my health; I saw others far worse off than myself and I felt I had to do something for myself. I had to get going again.

"Coming to the group and having some private counselling at The Foundation really helped me through. It was great to be able to share the problems and talk about them.

"My husband divorced me and has remarried. In 1985, I felt confident enough to buy a block of land and begin building my own house. It was a great therapy. Having to organize tradesmen, choose materials and fittings; it was a lot of hard work.

"My son and I lived seven months in a caravan — through the winter. We went through a lot, but now, with the house completed, we know we have achieved a lot.

"I continue to watch my diet and meditate. The meditation, which was not so good at the start, goes well for me now. I also walk a lot with our dog and enjoy my work. In fact, I am really happy and optimistic for the future."

Congratulations to Sylvia who has demonstrated that by facing a major life change, facing the challenges and dealing with them, a positive outcome and a happy, satisfying life can follow.

October 1987

Lynette Archer

Early in 1976 I went to the doctor because I was experiencing vague pains and irregularities in the bowel. Basic tests didn't reveal anything and the doctor felt it was psychological as I was working part-time and having to leave my three-year-old son with my sister.

Twelve months later Shane was born, but unlike the first pregnancy, this time it had been difficult. For several days after the birth I experienced excruciating abdominal pains. The cause couldn't be found so I took my baby home and the pain gradually subsided.

But there seemed to be a steady weight loss and occasionally the pains would return which eventually sent me back to the doctor and more tests. A barium meal and enema revealed some abnormality, so, on Friday 30th September, two weeks after my 30th birthday, taking my six month old son with me, I was admitted to hospital for more detailed investigation. The diagnosis: probable bowel cancer; the treatment: surgery the next Monday.

Mum was quick on the scene to help and I weaned Shane over that weekend. I had a good howl and wondered 'why me' and asked that family and friends not visit me as I felt I couldn't cope with their pity."

The surgery revealed extensive cancer of the bowel that had spread across onto the surface of the womb with spots near the liver and kidneys. The surgeon successfully removed the cancerous bowel and put a colostomy in place. He also performed a hysterectomy which included removing the ovaries.

I was told the colostomy was to be temporary and that it would be rejoined after six weeks. In fact it was three months later, but by then my doctor had confided that he really did not expect to be able to do it ever! I was told that only about 10% of people ever survive my type of situation.

Three weeks later I went home. Mum and Dad had moved in to help with the boys and together with my husband, the rest of the family gave great support.

Mum read everything she could get her hands on and started me on a good diet including plenty of fresh juices.

Soon after I started a seven week program of radiotherapy and each time I came home Mum would be waiting with another juice. I remember thinking: Oh no! If I have to have to swallow another green drink ... Sometimes it felt like the cure was worse than the complaint, but I felt I had to do it and the diet and juices certainly did the trick!

We found a G.P./naturopath who helped fine-tune the diet and offered other supportive treatments, and then it was on to eighteen months of chemotherapy which I handled extremely well. I didn't lose my hair, and the only side effect was a nauseous feeling like morning sickness for about an hour after each treatment. I'm sure, to a large extent, it was due to the good diet and juices I was on. And I had a very strong motivation in that I didn't want my children to grow up without their mother.

So we did a lot to help ourselves. When I had the colostomy closed, my G.P./naturopath persuaded the surgeon to add Vitamin C to my drip. I had the operation in the morning and in the afternoon I was jumping around, in my surgeon's words, 'like a schoolgirl'. That experience led to a close collaboration between the G.P. and surgeon, both for me and subsequent patients which was a very encouraging sign.

Twelve months after the diagnosis I was over the worst and the family was looking for a new venture. Based on our reading and experience we felt a need to promote a healthier way of eating so we began Apple-A-Day, a health food take-away shop. From small beginnings it mushroomed rapidly. We learned a lot more about how to prepare healthy food and we derived a lot of joy in knowing that we were offering a healthy alternative to the usual take away food.

Cancer was a learning experience for me. It forced me to look at my life and to re-evaluate my priorities, to find a meaning in whatever came my way and to learn from it. I can now see some of the habits I had that contributed to the cancer developing.

- Like always putting my own feelings and needs second and doing what I thought was expected of me, even if it was not what I wanted to do. That has its toll, done continuously.
- Like never expressing my emotions outwardly, particularly if I was upset or angry. I have now learned to say what's on my mind. (Most of the time anyway).
- Like wanting to change people and situations around me and becoming frustrated because it wasn't happening. I now realise I can only change myself and I try to accept others as they are, not how I want them to be.

I am convinced that illnesses are not just bad luck, that they happen for a reason. If you search for and find those reasons and make the changes, then you can start to rebuild your health.

January 1988

Footnote:

It is now seventeen years to the week since I was first diagnosed. I have remained in very good health, practising the sound principles put in place back then, particularly those of good nutrition and stress reduction. I have learned so much that I can truly say that it has been an amazing and a rewarding journey. Mum (Dorothy Edgelow) has continued to expand her knowledge of healthy eating habits and now runs the kitchen of The Gawler Foundation where they serve delicious, nutritious meals prepared with love.

September 1995

Eve Oakley

Eve Oakley attended the first ever 12 week program of the Melbourne cancer support group. It began on 14th September, 1981. At the time, Eve was battling an advanced brain tumor and secondary leukaemia.

In those first days we sat in rows like at a lecture. As Eve recalls, after the first two weeks everyone demanded to sit in a circle so that they could talk to each other more easily!

Eve has been through a remarkable amount in these last three years. At those first sessions, she appeared so sick, often she appeared n the verge of fainting or passing out. But she kept coming, became excited about the possibilities and forged ahead. Over the first year, it seemed there were several severe ups and downs. Yet each time Eve fought back, found the next step and moved on. Years passed and the cancer began to fade into memory. Then in 1985 came the tragic death of her 18-year-old daughter Jane. Eve had to battle the guilt of feeling her illness had denied her the opportunity of spending enough tim with her daughter. She recognised how easy it would have been to have given up and taken what seemed the easy way out, to let the stress of it all feed her disease and overwhelm her.

Eve determined to stay well. She did not want to think that her daughter's death could be blamed for her own. So Eve has had to face the grief and begin yet again.

Seven years later, Eve is an inspiration. Doubly. Firstly she overcame two supposedly terminal forms of cancer. Then she was faced with an incredibly stressful personal crisis. With the help of her family and friends and what she gained along the way, Eve is a truly remarkable survivor. Here she relates more of her story.

"It is now so long ago that I was sick that I can hardly remember when it was that I first came to see you; it must have been in 1981.

More than 10 years ago I was suffering from persistent headaches and dizziness. I was losing weight at an alarming rate. A cyst was removed from my right facial antrum and I was still very unwell when my husband went on study leave. We lived overseas for a year, in 1979. By that time the headaches had become more severe and my vision was blurred. In New York tests revealed that I had a cerebellar astrocytoma and I was told that it was inoperable and that the prognosis was very poor.

I was given chemotherapy, but after the fourth treatment I was feeling so sick and depressed that I discontinued the course. I strongly felt that my getting better was now beyond my control, as I was too weakened and helpless to .do anything for myself. Doctors subsequently diagnosed a leukemic condition, 'an unfortunate side-effect of the chemotherapy'. Tests revealed, however, that the tumor was shrinking. I found the tests intrusive and I was so depressed after the visits to the doctor that I decided I had to find another way of getting better. I was told by the doctor that without more treatment for the brain tumor I would have no longer than three months to live, whereas treatment would prolong my life for perhaps a year. I could not cope with that at the time.

Six months earlier, in England, I had followed a T.M. course and found that helpful in coping with the pain and the pressure in my head. When back in Melbourne I had the help from a friend who gave psychic healing and acupuncture and helped me to meditate. I then joined your classes and immediately realised that I was given a chance and the insight to do things for myself. It was great! This realisation that there really was a way of doing things for yourself, it was in your own hands. But I was feeling so lousy at the time it really was not easy. We were learning a lot, the group met at other times to talk more and everyone encouraged each other and drew on each other's strength. Diet, meditation, spiritual healing, psychiatric help, acupuncture, intensive vitamin C therapy, a visit to the healers in the Philippines, which provided me with much needed energy, and the tremendous trust and support I received from my husband and our friends, all contributed to my gradually getting better. It took a long time, though, not without its set-backs.

I have been feeling well and healthy and holding down a full time job for more than four years now. I helped in your support group until 1985 when my daughter Jane died. That was a time of crisis. Although the grief, after all this time, is still fresh, I am keeping healthy and I made a promise to the memory of Jane to not get sick again.

I do believe that my illness somehow was connected with a traumatic experience I had when I was 10 years old during the Second World War occupation of Holland and it was with the help of a psychiatrist while I was ill that I could confront that experience and talk about it for the first time since I was a child. I think that just about sums it up. I should perhaps mention that absolute bullet-proof single-mindedness was another factor that helped to get me better.

Rob Baird

As part of a super scheme medical examination in 1981, Rob Baird mentioned a wart-like lump on his left knee. Over the past few months, every time it had been knocked it seemed to bleed easily. The G.P. conducting the examination suggested quite casually that it be removed then and there. Surprisingly, the lump was not sent off for investigation.

The wound did not heal well, taking months to finally close over. Twelve months later, in June of 1982, Rob noticed an unusual lump in his left groin. This time a specialist's biopsy revealed that Rob had secondary melanoma. The advice was for surgery the next day.

"I was hesitant," Rob said. "I felt fine. Perhaps they had mixed the medical records." But this was no mistake. The surgery was carried out the next day. The lump, a lymph node, was removed, as were the chain of nodes up Rob's leg and past his groin. Also removed was a 10 cm area of skin around the knee — the sight of what was assumed to be the initial melanoma. While many of the other lymph nodes appeared blackened like melanomas often do, only the lump was confirmed as being infiltrated with secondary melanoma.

The surgeon did me the favour of saying that medical science had very little to offer melanoma patients. He said that there was a 70% chance of recurrence in five years."

"My immediate reaction was very depressed. I thought of myself as a realistic person. As an engineer you are taught to assume the worst: if you are building bridges you have to cover the worst possibility. So, I was reading the worst into this.

"Then a friend heard Ian speaking on the radio, and I joined the Melbourne cancer support group. It was a great benefit to meet other people with cancer, to share our problems and experiences in a friendly atmosphere and to encourage each other to continue along a path to good health. There was a weekly dose of enthusiasm from Ian and Grace. Also my wife Pru was so supportive, always seeing the positive side of my situation.

"The support group opened a lot of avenues for us all. Only a certain number were for me. Some held no interest, some did not work.

"Meditation had the most immediate effects. I had been so tense, it was a new experience to learn how to relax. I also had to learn where I fitted into the world. I needed to stop putting myself and close relationships last. I learnt to take life less seriously, I learnt to laugh, to watch the world go by and to enjoy living. I began to stop being upset by things that I could not change. For me, learning to cope with death and dying was a very important part of it.

"Early in 1983, I attended meditation with Ainslie Meares. Dr Meares was the manifestation of calm and tranquility. Burdens and troubles were always left at the door of "the quiet place", calm and stillness took their place.

"The summer after joining the group, I tried a 10 day grape fast, followed by slowly introducing the range of other foods — to determine if I had any food allergies or sensitivities. After one month, it appeared I was allergic to grapes! Subsequently, it was revealed that my body was sensitive to food combinations and I continued on a Pritikin-like maintenance diet.

"The support group was a real melting pot. Being politically aware and conscious of feminist views, it was particularly interesting to see the women in the groups changing. And changing so quickly. I noticed that very quickly they became more aware, more confident, more assertive. They stood up for themselves more. Those who were patients seemed to steam ahead of their husbands. Often it seemed as if the men were not used to being supportive. They had to learn how to do it, whereas the women did it more easily.

"When the men were the patients, they usually had a woman in the background. But these women kept up, it was not so hard for them to make changes and go with their partners as it was for the men support people.

"Often changes took place very fast. Relationships could come under a lot of stress. The men wanted things to be as they were before. But they never could be. The wives of men patients, however, would go with the changes and support their husbands.

"A lot of women patients had husbands expecting them to cook separate meals — on top of coping with their illness, the home and family. One lady patient even cooked three meals — one for herself, one for her husband and the other for the children! Finally she felt she had to have time to herself. She went on a holiday so that she could concentrate on her diet and other needs. It hurt her, but she knew she had to do it. Her husband was supportive in that he recognized she needed to go and he looked after the children while she was away. But like a lot of men he found it difficult to change himself. Many of the husbands seemed happy for their wives to go to the group as long as they did not upset the family routines!

"That lady did tremendously well. After a while the whole family adjusted and things generally got better.

I was fortunate. I had known Pru for seven years before my diagnosis. It made us realize that we could not live without each other. We made a commitment to each other and that cemented our relationship. We were married in 1983, our first child born in 1986, and now Pru is pregnant again. That has been fantastic. You don't realize what parenthood is until you are there, it's just amazing. It's good to look at the world through the eyes of a child. It simplifies everything. It relaxes you somehow and shows you how important life is.

"I am a different person now to what I was six years ago. I now lead my life one step at a time. I don't take on too much, I am aware of my limitations. As a result I am happier and more at peace. I feel that having cancer has been a tremendous learning period in my life. Even though I have relaxed my diet somewhat, the principles I learnt through the support group still guide my life.

not curing the condition which continued to deteriorate and disrupt every aspect of my life. I am a graphic designer by profession and an artist and calligrapher through emotional necessity.

Re-creation Retreat, Yarra Valley Living Centre: 19–24 November, 1991

I attended a 6-day meditation retreat run by Ian Gawler through a need to withdraw from my increasingly intolerable life situation — in particular the pain, discomfort and sheer frustration of my hand, wrist and forearm. The program consisted of good nutrition, yoga, massage therapy and a minimum of 4–5 hours meditation relaxation daily (meditating for health, insight, creative and spiritual development). This was combined with a retreat environment and caring and compassionate staff.

During the course of the week I underwent a spiritual and attitudinal healing which resulted in a total shift in perception and a public expression of emotion (grief). The ability to weep was something which I had been incapable of for 33 years.

The rest from my daily routine had not however alleviated the symptoms of my hand, wrist or forearm as I had hoped. If anything they were considerably aggravated yet I found myself able to cope far better than before, almost with a natural ease.

Consequences: 29th November, 1991

The days following my experience at the retreat were spent in a state of shock interspersed with bouts of uncontrolled and uncontrollable weeping as I both adjusted to my new perspective of reality and finally grieved for and released most of my past.

I was able to speak with my father for the first time without being intimidated by him and actually experienced some measure of peace in his presence. There is still some residual tension and ill feeling and this will have to be dealt with. I have not been able to totally forgive him.

My hand, wrist and forearm were now presenting me with unbearable pain which I could only partially relieve through meditation. In desperation I played a *Healing Journey* tape (a meditation exercise in guided imagery) by Ian Gawler and fell asleep still listening to it.

Two hours after awakening the next morning I was stunned by the realisation that not only had the swelling of my wrist lessened noticeably, but that I was free of any pain or discomfort as well — my condition was healed.

12th January 1992

I find myself experiencing no pain whatsoever from either my hand, wrist or arm — regardless of activity unless I regress (momentarily). Such a regression is marked by a sudden, sharp and painful return of symptoms, which can be removed through a conscious effort to relax and 'let go' of any emotional stress or physical tension which has developed. Mention of or concentration on my right arm will also bring about a dull pain.

As a consequence of my experiences over the past 14 months I find it a great pity that the medical profession chooses to concentrate on treating the physical symptoms of disease in isolation from the emotional, spiritual and psychological aspects.

I have always known — but rarely admitted — that disease is merely the outcome of mental attitude. Surely then it follows that if feelings and emotions can be dealt with, the disease will simply disappear.

October 1992

Claire

Claire had just finished 18 holes of golf when we spoke together. It was a different story just over 12 months ago when surgery had diagnosed a very rare cancer (in the Bartland's glands — the third case in the world!). Claire had been experiencing irritation for two years previously, but it had been dismissed as insignificant by her gynaecologist.

Now a second radical operation was recommended to remove the rest of the cancer and associated glands. But this would involve really mutilating changes, skin grafts and other secondary effects which was a very daunting prospect.

Claire has always been a determined lady. She worked for many years as a couturier in Collins Street before changing professions to become the first woman real estate agent on the Mornington Peninsula. After great initial opposition, she became very successful and was soon sales manager.

With specialists pressing her to go ahead with the surgery, Claire sought professional counselling. She was asked what she would do if she did only have three months to live — what were the 10 most important things she wanted to get done. "Writing the list out led to the main soul searching of my life. The thing that came first was that I really wanted to develop the spiritual side of my life — something I had neglected since a teenager. I set out to aim to find Faith and Trust in God.

"As the list progressed, I soon realised I did want to live not die and that I did not want the operation. I thought what difference does it make if I do go now or later. My husband died 11 years ago and I have no family, but I wanted to live and in one piece! I remember hearing that we are on this earth as a learning experience. So I determined to pull my socks up, to start living and take the cancer as just that — a learning experience."

As Claire worked on herself, she maintained visits to the specialist. Each time he implored her to have surgery — until November. "Then he was dumbfounded and hardly knew how to tell me that he was overjoyed with my condition."

Claire still has a little way to go but "I feel now it is full steam ahead for a complete recovery.

"I feel sure I recovered from a combination of things. The A.C.P.F. classes set me on the right track and I adhered to the meditation and diet. Being on my own left me feeling envious of others there with a support person in tow, but I got a lot of support from all the others. I never do things by halves and I stuck to it. I did develop Faith in the spiritual sense and importantly, I took personal responsibility for my condition. I realized and accepted that the stresses I had been under had caused the cancer and that having caused it, I could reverse it."

As proof of her optimism, Claire has just gone to great lengths to renovate her kitchen — well done!

Claire has asked for her surname to be left out but is happy to talk with and encourage other patients if you want to contact her via the office.

February 1986

Jackie Woodroffe

Jackie Woodroffe had one incredible day back in March 1983. In the morning she attended the funeral of a dear friend, who had died of cancer. In the afternoon she was diagnosed with breast cancer.

She was offered three choices by her surgeon: remove just the lump itself, have a mastectomy or have a biopsy and await the results. Although it was a large lump, a borderline case, Jackie opted for removing just the lump.

After the operation, the diagnosis was confirmed and five or six of 13 lymph nodes were affected. "I was just numb. I didn't know the ramifications; I knew they weren't good, I was just numb."

"The reactions of all around were so bad. There were tears in the nurses' eyes. I thought, 'This is it, I'm going to die, and in the not too distant future.' "

Jackie has three children and has been the very successful head of the migrant education department at the Footscray College of Technical and Further Education.

"Then I thought, 'I know that I can be strong and I certainly am determined.' So I began to question everyone on the self help options. The doctors said there was no empirical evidence to support it — only the medical treatment. They said you must have a positive attitude. I replied, 'Where is the empirical evidence for that!' "

"But I let them treat me the way they wanted to. I started chemotherapy. It was interrupted for some radiotherapy, then continued. Then it was interrupted again for a radio-isotope implant. By then I was so weak I could not take the anaesthetic. I had to be pre-meded three times before the anaesthetist was prepared to go through with it.

"Every time I went into hospital I had this feeling of everyone in there being worse off than me. Soon it was back to the chemo. In September of 1983 I heard of Ian's seminars, but thought I would just keep to the chemo.

"Towards the end of the treatments, the oncologist looked at the blood count, saw how low it was and said, 'We are not going to chase every little cancer cell.' These words really scared me and that treatment was half strength. The last treatment was full strength again and it really flattened me.

"Then I had a scan only to find there was cancer in five of my ribs. I was very upset and angry after all that treatment. The doctor said that there was nothing more they could do and that my prognosis was from six months to five years. I wanted to know.

"We had a holiday and I saw others that abused themselves and their lives. I thought how unfair it was, how can they do that and get away with it?"

Jackie came to the Melbourne cancer support group 12 weeks program in December 1983.

"I changed my life, my attitudes, became more positive. I started meditation and freed my life of the hurly burly. I switched to a strict vegetarian diet."

By May 1984 another scan showed only one rib affected and the most recent battery of tests in December 1986 were all clear.

Now Jackie says, "A lot of the time I forget that I am, or have been, a cancer patient. If I do get aches or pains, I can get down with it; however, then I do more meditation. But it does place an ongoing stress on relationships. Generally I feel fine but there are times when I get frustrated.

"Now I do spend quite a deal of time counselling friends and friends of friends." Jackie did spend a while giving valuable service on The Gawler Foundation committee. She has a very positive message to share with others.

July 1987

Dorothy Duncan

Dorothy Duncan is definitely exuberant. In typical fashion she says, "I'm not sure which applies — 'The old grey mare, she ain't what she used to be' or 'Wot the hell, wot the hell; there's life in the old girl yet!' "

Dorothy has been indulging a passion — tennis, practising with an 18-year-old youth. In December 1983, the mood was quite different. Then a biopsy of a breast lump was treated with great suspicion by her doctor, although it was three days before the positive diagnosis of cancer was confirmed.

"The initial reaction was panic. Really, you felt like you were looking possible death in the eyeball. You think of the family particularly, and how they will cope. I didn't cry; during the day no one knew or picked it up. The nights were the worst. Every so often you get this sweeping feeling of blind panic.

"After the three days I had it sorted out and had prepared myself. Surgery was recommended immediately, but I wanted to make sure it had not spread and insisted on scans. These were clear, but after the surgery it was found that two lymph nodes were affected.

"The surgeon described the cancer as 'a virulent little bastard!' and wanted me to have chemo. I took hours of convincing as I was concerned about depressing my immune system. The doctor convinced me I had no other choice so I began a 12 month course.

"It was hell. The worst year of my life. I managed to keep working, just taking five days off each month. But it was not just how sick it left you feeling, but the other things with the body. I guess I do resent it in many ways, because of the changes which took place, that I think I am stuck with. With the premature menopause, the hot flushes, the loss of taste and smell, and the hypersensitivity to some things; aerosol sprays still nearly make me throw up.

"I guess I kept going for the children mostly. At first all the family were keen for me to have it, but after three months they wanted me to stop. I felt I had committed myself and told myself it was going to work, so I stuck with it. It was the hardest bloody 12 months of my life!

"However, it was really quite humbling through all this to become aware of the incredible number of people who were so caring. It made me more aware of what makes the world go around.

Twelve months of chemotherapy completed, Dorothy then discovered that she had cervical dysplasia. "I overheard it actually, at the doctors. It seems they didn't tell me at the first sign three months earlier, as they didn't want to worry me! At the second test the affected area was clearly visible.

"It was then I thought I had to do something for myself. I had always believed in the power of the mind, but was unsure of how to use it. So I began by talking to this area and pretty simply told it to go away. Attending the 10-day residential program really gave me the tools to work with although by then the dysplasia had cleared anyway."

Now Dorothy is very interested in the whole concept of self help programs. She finds that she gets a lot of calls from friends and strangers, wanting to talk to her.

Dorothy has a teaching gift, working with the Special Education Unit, visiting regional schools and children with learning and emotional difficulties. Demanding work. She also is involved in the newly established Horsham Cancer Support Group being run through the local hospital, as well as conducting a small meditation group at home.

"In one sense I feel I want to help as much as I can. Often my friends ask if I mind with all these people calling? Not at all — I want to do as much as I can; but it does mean that it is not easy to get away from the cancer thing. There are times when you need to just get away and do something else.

"I also find that meditating before a group session is a great help. The job too is physically tiring and emotionally demanding. If I get tired, I know I get problems. It is very important to keep yourself on an even keel. I do that with meditation, diet and attitude. The meditation helps with the kids too. After a good session in the morning, even a little monster can't touch you, try as they might!"

For Dorothy then, cancer has brought a new perspective to life. "In the long term it has led to a sorting out of priorities. I now appreciate people more and see things through different eyes. You appreciate the country even more, spend time to look at something. A simple thing that is really beautiful. It's a heightening of awareness. Things that you were vaguely aware of before, took for granted in fact, are now so wonderful.

"Relationships have changed a bit. I am less inclined to let others organise my time for me now. I am much more aware of the value of time and my need to control it.

"And I am probably less tolerant of crap! — you know from other people. I either avoid it or am more direct. Say what I think and express my opinion more. I am not so prepared to compromise myself, to put up with it."

It seems that not only has Dorothy learnt a lot through this experience, she is giving a great deal back as well!

July 1987

Wendy Hill
Overcoming Rheumatoid Arthritis

I received this letter from Wendy and reproduce it to show how our principles of living well, living to the full, can make such a difference:

"I am 29 years old and have had rheumatoid arthritis for five years. After the birth of my first child it became more and more severe. There were countless trips to the hospital for treatment and, looking back, it only provided a little temporary relief.

Although I knew the doctors and staff were doing their best for me, the endless waiting at the hospital for appointments, constantly being around sick people, the extra effort needed to carry the baby around, and to drive the car, did nothing to improve my condition.

I'd been told that flare-ups can occur anytime and that there was really very little that could be done except to treat the symptoms and hopefully slow down the rate of joint degeneration.

After two years I became very depressed and took Tofranil for six months. I began to ask myself why I got this disease and what was happening to my body. The more books I read the more I felt the answers were within myself and that the arthritis was the end result of many things which had happened in my life. It was my body's way of reacting to stress and trying to adapt to living in this materialistic physical world.

I decided that I was definitely not relying on other people or foreign chemicals for the rest of my life. My health was my responsibility. So I gradually stopped my hospital treatment and cut my pills down to two aspirin occasionally.

I became pregnant again, stopped working and enjoyed an improvement in health. Two days after the birth of my son everything crashed down again. The pains came back and I couldn't even pick up the baby or change his nappies. Even a simple thing like sitting up in bed meant that each movement had to be planned. Over the next three months the arthritis became more severe and deep depression set in again. I could hardly move as I was in so much pain and just felt like sleeping and lying in bed all day long. I'd read that hell literally meant "isolation" and I think that I must have been there. I cut myself off from the outside world and from my family to some extent. It didn't make sense because there was every reason for me to live — two wonderful children, a loving and supportive husband, and a comfortable home. Yet I felt as if my body was being slowly drained of all its energy and was such a burden to me. I had read that the difference between arthritis and cancer was that one can kill you and the other can make you wish you were dead. And I wanted to die.

I still refused to take any medication except occasional aspirin, and remembered seeing a T.V. documentary about your story, Ian, and also a newspaper article several years earlier. My doctor gave me your phone number and wished me well with it. He didn't seem very hopeful though.

When I'd stopped treatment earlier I'd known what sort of help I didn't want, but hadn't thought about what I should do instead. This is where you came in.

Within two weeks of the support group course I had started a diet, was meditating and trying to develop a more positive attitude by repeating affirmations each day. Miracles didn't happen overnight, but over about six–eight weeks I had lost weight, was feeling lighter and more energetic, could get some sort of enthusiasm about things and even see as far as the next day. I could even laugh more easily.

Now after three and a half months I am much calmer with the children, am very relaxed, and am getting some ideas for next year when I hope to start a bit of work again.

Having arthritis has forced me to slow down, look at my life, ask who I am and where I'm heading. I would not have done these things otherwise.

For so long I'd concentrated on the pain and problems of the disease that I'd lost a sense of perspective on my life in general. Now I can move much more smoothly and freely and am very relaxed. I even gave my four year old daughter a whizzy the other day. I am not looking so aged and bent as I used to and my complexion has cleared up considerably. Mentally I have improved out of sight. There is a deeper feeling of happiness and inner contentment, and more of a spiritual awareness.

There is still a long way to go but I know I'm on the right path now. Thank you so much Ian for showing me how to find a peace of mind and better health not only for me, but for my family too.

I'm so much happier now and feel as if I'm starting all over again and have a bright future.

Once again, many many thanks. Your support groups should not just be for people with cancer, but for everyone."

October 1985

Neil Sambell

Grace and I first heard from Neil Sambell when we were living in Adelaide back in 1978. He told us later that his half page typed letter requesting help had taken him half an hour to complete, typing with one finger.

Neil began to take an active role in his disease which by then was well advanced. A little over a year later came the first hand written letter. It was in 1982 that Neil called on us in Yarra Junction to tell us with great excitement of his completion of a five km bushwalk at Wilson's Promontory.

Neil is happy to share his experiences with other Multiple Sclerosis (M.S.) patients and can be contacted via the office. Here we include his advice:

Factors Significant in My Experience With M.S.

The following approach is no guarantee for success with M.S., but I feel it was partly (if not largely) responsible for my continued reversal.

Creation of the Healing Environment:

I believe that one cannot continue with one's previous life pattern (in which, it should be noted, the disease took root), but that it was necessary to create the healing environment — both internally (mentally, spiritually and physiologically) and externally.

The previous life style had to be replaced by a simple, peaceful, aesthetic, positive, but purposeful life. It is important that one be at peace and guilt-free for where there is peace, there is healing.

Therefore, it follows that one must look at the healing process as one package and not isolated practices. Techniques are complementary to each other.

Diet:

The evidence indicates that diet definitely has a beneficial effect on the long-term course of the M.S. The principles outlined in the book, *The Multiple Sclerosis Diet Book* by Professor Roy L. Swank are neurologically supported. His theories are substantiated by a trial of his diet conducted with M.S. patients over a period of between 29 and 35 years.

Exercise and Rest:

In his book: *Multiple Sclerosis — Control of the Disease*, W. Ritchie Russell (also a former Professor of Neurology) writes: "For those who have the persistence and enthusiasm necessary to carry out the program advised, the future course of the M.S. is likely to become **benign**".

I was fortunate to be able to lead a peaceful life style, to have sufficient rest and to avoid traumatic situations. Fitness and general health were (and still are) very important.

Medical Help:

I hold in high esteem and cooperated fully with the medical profession, although some do not fully understand all my attitudes and activities.

Divine Healing and Power of the Mind:

The power of the mind cannot be overstated. For me, this is interrelated to spiritual attitudes and faith. The belief that the matter is improving steadily (even though it may be unnoticeable in the short-term) is bolstered by all the other avenues. One should positively act on this belief, but always staying within one's limits.

St. Joseph's, Northcote's weekly charismatic prayer group was invaluable — for their regular prayers and in helping me gain and maintain a healthy and positive mental attitude.

I believe and expect that God's miracles and healings are part of reality, but there does not seem to be any consistency here. However, miracles do frequently occur. Some people are particularly gifted by God as being channels for God's healing power. I sought these out and am especially indebted to (the late) Mrs. Mary Rogers. Many prayers were said over me, many spiritual insights were gained and I met some wonderful people. I did not aggressively fight the disease, but gave it over to God, peacefully prayed and sought prayer. I also literally applied James 5, 13–14.

Other Matters:

Philippine healing has some amazing testimonies despite adverse publicity — but I do not understand the spiritual implications.

I owe special thanks to Ian and Grace Gawler for introducing me to many of the above factors and for their support, particularly when the M.S. was active.

February 1986

Joan Simpson

Joan Simpson will be known to many, Queenslanders especially, who have heard her inspiring views regarding cancer as an opportunity for personal growth. It certainly has, and continues to be, just that for Joan.

Joan discovered a breast lump which was confirmed to be cancerous in December 1982. She refused a mastectomy and just had the lump removed. This was followed with 30 days of radiotherapy.

At the time, Joan had just returned from a period living in the U.S. "I had worked as a receptionist/assistant in an holistic medical clinic there and had seen many people getting well. My marriage had collapsed in America and when I came back to Australia, deep inside, I really wanted to die. I couldn't do it directly to myself and it was as if the cancer would do it for me.

"However, once I had the surgery and began radiation, I was getting pretty cross with myself for wanting to die — just because someone else didn't think I was good enough!

"So I began using meditation, active visualisation, and vitamin and mineral supplements.

"Because I only had the lump out, I had a heavy treatment schedule. Yet despite the warnings of pain and other side effects, I was the only one of the ten ladies who went through with me, who had no problems.

"For the first time, this caused me to begin to feel that I could have some power over my own life. That was really exciting! Since then, however, there have been some lapses in faith. 18 months after the surgery, in 1984, a nodule appeared on my thyroid. I requested one month to work on it and sure enough it decreased. Now if I get stressed, up it comes. Intensify the efforts, regain the balance, down it goes. I seem able to control it.

"Another one was lumps in the neck. I didn't believe they were cancer and read how mercury poisoning from amalgam dental fillings could be involved. Well, I changed the amalgams and since then — no more swellings."

In April 1983, with Dr. Ruth Cilento, Joan initiated a cancer support group at the Relaxation Centre, Brisbane. An Ian Gawler seminar at the centre followed soon after and Joan soon had a new role as group leader. She has had patients live in her home, worked with other doctors and run residential programs.

"I loved it. It was inspiring for me, and it gave me confidence. A miracle had occurred for me in that cancer had led to my own attitudes changing. I could now help by presenting other new patients with options, but I felt my job was to inspire them to find answers within themselves.

"This work kept me going, gave me a purpose and a sense of worth. I learnt to handle the emotional side of it, mostly because I believe death is not the end and can see any suffering as only temporary.

"I came to know that those who faced death and saw it as a new beginning could let go and have a good death. It concerns me that society often feels shame in not fighting for life. Sometimes people do fight to the last and die badly. There can be a need to let go, and I use meditation and prayer to seek guidance as to what is required to help; when you really do care and are prepared to love someone, it does make a big difference.

"I still do cry with patients sometimes, but in a different way now. Sometimes I just feel a need to cry with people. I guess it's an empathic thing, talking and being sympathetic."

Now, nearly five years later, "the thought of cancer keeps me working on myself and my limitations. My mother often told me as a child that she wanted to die. I picked it up and have had trouble getting over it fully and maintaining the joy of life which I feel so strongly at times. It has been a strong emotional habit to break.

"Now I pray a lot; I could not have made it without prayer. At the moment I want to work on myself. I am in a conventional job and my husband is back in my life. I am learning a lot about male/female relationships.

"I believe I got cancer in the breast because I was not nurturing myself. When my children were young I used to have these horrible nightmares. I was suckling this thin, wretched, whimpering child who had a smelly nappy on and appeared so uncared for. I could never understand it, as I gave everything I had to my children. Only recently when I was sick did I realise that the child was myself.

"Now I don't flagellate myself. I can accept myself and where I am at. I continue to meditate and get closer to my spiritual self. I aim to change slowly. I have good days and bad ones, mostly good. But being bright, bouncy Joany every day is bloody hard work!

"Cancer has pointed me in the right spiritual direction. I have learnt how the mind does control the body. The material and worldly things have become less important, although I still love to dress up. I have met and shared with so many people, that I have a better perspective. I see behind the facades and have much more understanding.

"I have learnt of the unimportance of death — it's what leads up to it that counts. But I also believe that death as a conscious experience is very important — especially if it is a part of living.

"I guess I am full of wise words now; how it will be at the time, we will have to wait and see!"

Joan has always impressed me by being really awake and alive. Interested, compassionate, caring, loving and inspiring, so many people have benefitted and continue to do so, through her presence.

July 1987

Mary Hunter

The thing that impresses me most about Mary is that here is a quietly spoken, gentle and loving lady who exudes a positive and confident air. She is very much at ease with herself and life in general, cares greatly for those around her and wants to actively share that concern.

Mary's first close contact with cancer came back in 1961 when her husband developed cancer of the bowel and liver. It was a time when there was a great deal of fear of cancer and the subject was "pushed under the carpet". It made Mary very angry that no-one would talk of it and, worse, she was advised to tell her husband he merely had an ulcer. He suspected more and finally was told that his surgery had in fact removed all his cancer — "walk out, forget and don't tell anyone".

Mary did not question it at the time — she felt his doctors knew best and it was all right to go along with the deception. When a relapse came and the liver was affected, hepatitis was the story.

Mary has two adult daughters. Kim is a nurse specialising in coronary care and Keryn is on an invalid pension following a bad accident seven years ago. Mary has been working as a machinist, designing and making samples of frocks and other clothes.

In 1979 Mary had a superficial complaint checked only to be diagnosed as having cancer herself. She was deeply shocked and underwent six weeks of further tests which relieved her by concluding it was not cancer after all! In 1981 the condition reoccurred and Mary had treatment for cancer of the vulva. Also, she had suffered stomach ulcers twice before and these pains had re-occurred, so while under anaesthetic, her stomach was examined. Cancer of the stomach was diagnosed also and at a subsequent operation two thirds of her stomach was removed. A scan showed cancer in her liver and a number of lumps appeared in her neck and shoulders.

Mary was told she could not expect to live for more than 18 months, but was back at work three months after her operation! She had three months of chemotherapy in 1981, but then declined more treatment as, in her words, "I honestly felt I could do a better job myself. I decided I was just going to live my life doing the best I could. If God wanted to take me, He would — if not, OK."

Setting out to paint the roof of her house, Mary also decided to save for regular holidays as treats. She is currently working on a big aim — "Hong Kong for Christmas!"

"I have learnt a lot," says Mary, "not to panic and not to get stressed. My doctor says I did the right thing for me in stopping the treatment, but he says I can always come back if I want to." Mary has had two scans since her surgery and speaks very highly of her treatment at the Royal Melbourne Hospital and of her doctor's care. She says her last test showed her blood is "the best it has ever been."

In early 1984 a friend showed Mary an article on Ian and she said, "He must have had a strength I could never have and besides I just couldn't face the idea of the diet!" Then Keryn enthused her and in May 1984 she began an A.C.P.F. program. She was accompanied by Kim and together they have gradually changed onto the maintenance diet (which Mary is now a great advocate for), developed a daily practice of meditation and built up more confidence and positivity. Mary feels that she is still getting better every day.

Having seen the negative effects of the fear of cancer causing havoc with her husband twenty years ago, Mary is keen to do all she can to allay those fears and replace them with positive, constructive attitudes.

Mary, you are an inspiration to us all.

December 1984

Judith Tregear

A year ago last Friday, in February of 1988, I had my brain tumour surgically removed. All went well and everyone was very relieved. However, I developed post-operative complications — pulmonary embolus (blood clots) — and ended up spending the whole of the month of February in hospital.

The neurosurgeons had not been able to put my cranial bone back after the removal of the tumour, because there was too much swelling. I went home, on a course of anti-coagulation drugs for three months, minus a rather large piece of my frontal bone.

Waiting to go back into hospital, trying to cope with shock, pain, sadness and terrible fear, I felt very alone at times, even though I was supported by my loving family and friends, and one exceptionally caring doctor from the Royal Melbourne.

Right from the beginning of my hospitalisation I had known instinctively that my attitude was of crucial importance. When I temporarily lost confidence (during the complications), I had to struggle to regain my faith that everything would work out. There was no possibility of pretending to myself — I had to really believe.

At home there were different challenges. I was terrified of going back into surgery, afraid I would die, despite assurances that the bone replacement operation would be "a piece of cake". The operation to remove the tumour, although certainly life-saving, had also been rather drastic and violent. I cried a lot. In April my doctor suggested that I contact the Australian Cancer Patients Foundation.

I had a long talk to Stephen Taylor on the phone. I told him that I was afraid and very anxious, and that I felt as if my life spark was flickering and growing faint. Also that I was in a total crisis of belief. Almost the only thing I knew was that I wanted, 100% to live. He understood, and seemed to think it was natural for me to be feeling like this. It was a relief to talk with him, particularly as he himself had personal experience of major illness.

I returned to hospital, survived the second operation (of course), and came home in June with my bone back in its rightful place. In September I started the 12 week cancer patients support group at the Melbourne Living Centre, with my brother, Richard, as my support person. It was quite a decision to do the course; one thing I was anxious about was being in a room full of sick cancer patients, some of them terminal.

How depressing, how threatening. As we discovered on the last day of the course, we had all felt worried about this! What a relief to find that everybody was perfectly normal and nice! If there was any difference between the people in that room and those in "the rest of the world", it was that they were braver than we are generally required to be, because they were confronting one of the most undermining and difficult life situations — serious illness.

I found meditation difficult; an unquiet mind, my body in a bit of a state, problems with the progressive muscle relaxation exercise. I was quite tense and anxious. But I persevered, partly through determination and partly because I somehow always knew that it was deeply beneficial and healing. For the first three months at least I had frightening images of blood and violence, especially around my head. For months I had horrible dreams every time I went to sleep. Towards the end of the 12 week course I started to have visions of myself dying while meditating. A friend suggested I give up meditation immediately and see a psychiatrist. Ian Gawler talked with me about fear and control. He said that if I felt able to allow the fears to come and not fight or resist them, but to just let them run their course, they would eventually go. This is working!

After some relatively peaceful weeks again I began to experience graphic visions of brain surgery while meditating. As February 1989 approached, overflowing with "anniversaries" of C.A.T. scans, diagnosis, surgery etc. I felt quite upset. I have definitely made some progress in simply allowing these things to come and go, without getting completely overwrought. When Friday arrived, the anniversary of my operation — and I have felt all along that on some level my life began when I woke up from that first anaesthetic — I awoke very early and went through it all again in my mind, everything that happened this time a year ago. I couldn't help it. But instead of feeling distressed at some of the upsetting memories I found that all I could feel was joy. Joy and gratitude, that I am here now!

Through my involvement with the A.C.P.F. I have received not only support, but also inspiration. This is so important. It's wonderful to find that you can be strong and brave while in hospital. You don't forget what you learn in that situation. But coming home, looking at getting well, trying to find your life again, these challenges can be very daunting, particularly as they are long-term. I have improved marvellously, and have been extremely fortunate. When I look back over everything that has happened it all seems quite miraculous. But I still get frustrated and angry at the painful slowness and unevenness of recovery, still finding the major lessons of patience, acceptance and faith very difficult at times. The other day someone handed me a little book — "The reward of patience is patience" leapt off the page at me. I had to groan, and laugh!

After I came out of hospital I felt as if I had new eyes. Trees, birds, water, sky — all were freshly beautiful and clear. I felt very glad to be alive and intensely aware of the beauty and sacredness of all life. I was so able to appreciate the amazing lovingness of the people around me. It was as if a thin veil which had been between me and reality had been lifted. Now, although not yet fully fit, I feel happier and healthier than I ever have. Discovering that I want to live, totally, has been the most affirming experience of my life.

The latest development has surprised me — I am actually starting to enjoy meditating! I am finding it deeply restoring and restful and find myself going off to meditate even when I don't "have" to. It is certainly the single most important and helpful thing I am doing. My mother thinks that my recovery really got started when I did the 12 week course and began to meditate.

For many months I felt that everything in my life had been violently torn from me, and from my control, except for my choice of response. At times it seemed that most of the last year was just waiting, fear and loss. Now I know that right now is the most wonderful time of my life, and I can feel that I am finding my path. I am frequently reminded of one of my favourite sayings from zen macrobiotics, *"The bigger the front the bigger the back"*.

Yesterday some friends came to visit and we went and flew a kite near the water. It was a beautiful kite, and I felt as if I was meditating as I watched it soaring and diving, hovering and floating against the blue sky and the white clouds.

April 1989

Katie Prineas

In May 1988 Katie was diagnosed with non-Hodgkins lymphoma. She attended a 10-day residential program in June, 1989. In July 1992 she attended the follow-up course at the Yarra Valley Living Centre.

"In May 1988 I was diagnosed with one of the non-Hodgkins Lymphomas. (I believe there are about 300 different kinds of Lymphomas.)

"The doctor was not exactly sure which one I had at the beginning, but was quick to tell me that I could begin to haemorrhage at any time and that I had beween three months to three years to live.

"After leaving his surgery I sat in my car and thought about my sister and two of my best friends who had died of lymphomas and thought there is no way that I could put my husband and children through seeing me die like that. I also wanted to die with dignity and not to go through the pain and suffering my sister and friends went through.

"I thought there must be something that I can do, so I drove straight to a book shop and bought everything I could see on cancer.

"After reading *You Can Conquer Cancer* by Ian, I knew that there was hope and that I could do something to help myself.

"In June 1989 I did the 10-day live-in program and came home with lots of enthusiasm to meditate three times per day for one hour, exercise, juices and a very strict diet.

"My husband encouraged and supported me by growing wheatgrass and juicing it for me. The times I weakened and had no energy my daughter pushed me to swim and to be positive that I could lick this.

"I was so busy doing all these things I forgot about having a good time and living. All I was doing was cancer.

"Then in November 1990 my haemoglobin dropped down to below four. I was put into hospital and given three bags of blood every three to four days for three weeks as the cancer was knocking out the red cells as quickly as they were giving it to me. Also against my wishes and to please my family I had chemo every day for 21 days plus 75 mg of Prednisolone daily. By the end of December I was skin and bone. I could not walk and had pain that was humanely unbearable due to the side effects of the chemo. I was critically ill and the doctor did not give me any hope. I thought if I am going to die I would like to die at home. I stopped the chemo (the doctor said I would surely die), I was dying anyway.

"With the training of my 10-day program, I put into motion anything I was capable of doing. Especially letting go, meditating and using the pain control techniques.

"I was determined not to have drugs so that I could be aware of what exactly I was feeling. I raised a temperature of 39 to 40 for three weeks and spent most of the time in a cold bath day and night.

"Thanks to the wonderful support of my family, a few close friends and a wonderful naturopath I started slowly to get better.

"It took me three months of meditation, juices, exercise, swimming, balanced diet and lots of vitamin C, plus vitamins and minerals that my body needed to be able to even have the strength to drive my car.

"Today I am strong and happier than I have ever been in my life.

"When I was diagnosed with cancer I had no balance in my life.

"I have just completed the five day follow-on course. It was so strong and powerful as all of us in the group knew where we were at.

"Ian, Grace, Bob and Trevor were able to teach us on a more advanced level. There is so much more I have learnt about cancer and myself.

"I can honestly say that getting cancer has changed my whole outlook on life. I am now enjoying every day.

"When you are planning your life don't forget to put in the fun."

October 1992

Kay Chandler

In May 1986 a mastectomy was performed on me because of breast cancer, followed by five months of chemotherapy.

By May 1987 I was suffering physical problems with my back, hips and right leg. A scan showed that my breast cancer had spread to eleven parts of my body.

At the point of breaking the news to me, my doctor and husband were devastated — I too of course. However at that moment I felt that I did have another chance even though medically nothing could be done for me at that time. I decided to take the drug Tamosapen which I was told sometimes controls breast cancer for a time, and "believe" that it was helping me.

I also had something else to hold on to — it was "hope". I had just finished reading Ian Gawler's book *You Can Conquer Cancer* and whilst I was reading it, I began to have more and more faith in what he was saying. It made complete sense. When I received news that my cancer had spread I adopted his program straight away. Meditating for three hours per day, diet and working on all aspects of positive thinking, I put my "faith" in this program.

I also had my "faith" in God, and looking back, I was actually clinging to him during that traumatic time of sorting myself out. I had security.

Because I wanted to live so badly, I knew that I had to have enough "faith" in myself in being able to persevere in overcoming my cancer — making sacrifices and never giving up on my healing.

A month later — June 1987, my husband Reg and I attended a 10-day workshop in Victoria with Ian and his team and we weren't disappointed. It was the experience of our lives. We learned how to turn the tables on my disease and Reg has always been so thankful that he was able to come with me. He learned how to be supportive and understanding in our quest to conquer cancer. He has shared my cancer.

When we came home to Sydney we felt we needed continued inspiration in healing so I attended a stress management course for cancer patients at "Hillview", Turramurra. Also, because of my strong "faith" in God, I started attending the weekly Healing Service at St. Andrews Cathedral on Wednesday evenings. There I found a new power. In his sermons and through his books Canon Jim Glennon taught me how to combine the power of God with the same advice as Ian's — positive thinking, love, forgiveness for myself and others, and getting rid of resentments and hurts in one's life. I found that my meditating and working with God on any issues or problems in my life gave me the answers. It took patience and perseverance and self-honesty. It was so rewarding when I found that I had accomplished complete inner peace and contentment. There were no hurts or resentments, anxiety or stress — just love, peace and joy.

Because of these healing emotions my immune system was strengthening with each new wonderful day.

Persevering with my diet was not only building up my body, but it gave me a nice secure feeling of healing. I learned to condition my subconscious mind with healing thoughts and activities all day, every day — again building up my immune system.

Five months after attending Ian's workshop I had another scan which showed that much of my cancer had gone. At that stage, which is now twelve months ago, I still had some physical problems. However since then I have become physically strong and mentally confident. I've learned to have great power over my mind and to have enough "faith" in God to hand over my burden of cancer. This has taken away anxiety and replaced it with security, peace, joy and inner calm.

My daily affirmations of "Every day in every way I'm getting better and better" had come true.

Now I am not at all afraid of death and I think that the knowledge that my death is going to be wonderful (whenever) is really a life-giving thought.

I am still waiting for another scan which I know will be good, but it really doesn't matter to me any more, because through meditation, prayer, positive thinking and diet I have become very strong in controlling my health and my life — it's a new life!

I would like to share with you my first exercise in positive thinking for each day.

The moment I open my eyes in the morning, I allow God to hand me the day. Every morning I receive this beautiful gift of today and inside this gift are other gifts of joy, loads of love, understanding, patience, security, perseverance and power of mind. Because I am so lucky to receive this gift of today and "life", I promise that I will enjoy it and handle whatever comes my way in a calm, loving and positive way. If I continue to do this I know that the tomorrows will just keep coming.

I learned very early that if I was to move this mountain that it would be easier for me if I was to appoint myself a healing team and draw on them for strength and support. To be a member of my team one had to be a positive person and have "faith" (or believe) in everything that I was doing. It was headed by my husband Reg, my daughter and son and other family members. Also Ian Gawler, Canon Glennon, neighbour Pat, and my confidante Jenny Figtree who has given me constant and untiring support every step of the way during these last seventeen months.

I can only say that it's been a very rewarding adventure and experience, and most of all I want to say that anyone can do it if they really want to. I am just an ordinary everyday person, and if I can do it so can you if you have the need.

I took this road to healing simply because I read a book called *You Can Conquer Cancer.* Thank you Ian and Grace.

(Kay's scans in 1989 did in fact show her cancer almost completely gone.)

April 1989

Mary's Story written by Mark

Dear Ian,

I felt the need to write to you to let you know of the death of Mary, and also to give your group sessions some feedback from my perspective.

Mary's condition began to gradually deteriorate in July. She died on the 11th of December, but in spite of her extreme disabilities (due to back and leg pain, and later swelling) managed to remain active until two weeks before her death. When I think of the manner in which she/we managed during that period of time, I think very much of the acceptance of the need for quality of life and the undeniable power of positive thinking. Mary was a woman with great courage and determination. Many of the discussions raised in the group sessions (and subsequent discussions together and with others) gave us both a great many supportive ideas to focus on.

When I think back to my involvement with the group sessions (and I believe I can also speak for Mary on this), there are many issues that were raised and discussed that I feel helped me greatly during the whole process of Mary's initial recovery and then gradual deterioration.

The sessions and material on meditation and diet were the focus on which from the non-medical aspect, we were able to commence Mary's recovery. The meditation has continued to help me greatly in times of trouble. The diet which I still maintain to a reasonably successful degree helped immensely in terms of both our general health, but particularly (I believe) with regard to Mary's minimal sickness during her chemotherapy treatment period.

I know that the discussions around the concept of quality of life greatly supported our own thoughts, and we maintained a very active and happy life-style.

The ideas raised through discussion about death and dying were most supportive and encouraging. Mary and I were able to communicate freely (when her death became the obvious conclusion to her condition). Mary was able to die at home, and I (and many friends) shared the honor of being able to nurse her through that period. The satisfaction of being able to carry out such an important request is one that I will always value highly. Also, with regard to my own "recovery" from Mary's death, I feel these sessions have helped. I can remember being greatly saddened during the "death and dying" session. However, having had an opportunity to discuss some of those issues and then consider my attitude to dying has made Mary's absence easier in some respects at least. I think that I would like to attend another of the "death and dying" sessions, and would appreciate it if you could let me have a copy of the program that is currently running. I hope that things are running smoothly for you.

April 1986

Stephen Taylor

1981 is a good year to start. Four years previously my first marriage had broken up. I had taken on a new principal teacher's job, and moved house. My left side seemed weak and there were some other vague symptoms. After a visit to a bone specialist and then a neurologist, I was informed that 'I had minimal childhood hemiplegia. I was 98% OK, take it easy and it should be alright. And don't run the marathon.'

Not surprisingly, I took the last bit as a challenge, trained steadily and did it. Also I had started an organic garden, a new relationship and marriage; life was stable and flowing; I felt happy.

Then in 1982 we moved again and began to build a house and establish a farm from a bare paddock, in the Adelaide hills.

The Deputy Principal's position was demanding, so was the training for A-grade football umpiring and then my daughter's birth. So many new projects. I felt that whatever I wanted I could achieve. Every new idea I had I took on. All good projects, but so much of it.

Suddenly, in June 1985, it all came to a head. My left side became weak and after our 12–14 km runs, I could not lift my left arm. I had a worrying cyst on one finger also, so I went to the doctor to get it checked out.

Firstly, I was told I should have been checked yearly since 1981. Referred immediately to a neurologist, a C.A.T. scan showed a problem. It was centrally located, difficult to biopsy, perhaps it was a tumour! More tests over several months remained inconclusive. Finally came an angiogram. In the middle of this, my second marriage broke up and I had a strong urge to leave teaching.

Now I was told it was almost certainly a tumour! The nurse cried as I was told, but I felt my own emotions close over. At the same time there was this sense of relief in finally knowing what the problem was.

In retrospect, I recognize a part of me that sensed that I now had a socially acceptable excuse to let go of all that activity. What a relief! I had been feeling like I was trying to climb mountains all day. Not really knowing what mountain I was on, or why I was climbing. Getting to the top of one, feeling momentary satisfaction, then swinging on in search of the next peak. There was something awful inside of me driving me almost to destruction. A feeling of emptiness inside — while the outside was being filled with materialistic achievements.

At last it seemed like the tumour would allow me to let go of the striving. The feeling was relief — but in the same moment the old pattern left me with a feeling of guilt — the guilt of not doing, not achieving.

Then another month of tests with top neurologists. By November I was informed that 'a biopsy being inadvisable, to the best of our knowledge, it is a cystic astrocytoma. It is probably inoperable, chemotherapy is ineffective, we could try radiotherapy possibly.' We all decided to wait and observe it.

I went to try a homeopath and hypnotherapist. The neurologist told me not to waste my money, that he did not recommend them. I felt I got some help and then enquired of Ainslie Meares. 'Stephen,' said the neurologist, 'let's not hear anything more about faith healers.' It was not just the words, but the patronising way in which they were said that made me really angry. It was like he was taking my hope away.

So I went to Ainslie Meares in early March 1986, for four weeks. I lived in a tent in a caravan park, went to the meditation sessions and read and read. I felt like his books were written about me. The sadness overcame me, I started to let go of the guilts and then started to cry again.

Then there were new discoveries. It was all a deep and profound personal experience. It felt like in the meditation I had come home. I realized that there was an inner world and I rediscovered two words — love and God. I felt them, I came closer to them, but could still not even say them out loud to another person. Those four weeks changed the course of my life profoundly.

When I got back to Adelaide, I read Ian's book, went to a weekend seminar with Ian and Grace and then came to Melbourne for a residential program.

The residential program gave me the momentum to make the necessary changes in my life. At the same time there was a spiritual awakening in my life. I had partly learnt already to deal with the word 'love', now it was time to find out about God.

Back in Adelaide, I enrolled in the voluntary counselling course for the Adelaide support group. A lot of energy went into my lifestyle and getting well. I began counselling other patients, became much closer to my family and my father was learning how to hug! I attended many workshops and lectures and went back to my teaching job. I tried to re-establish the last marriage, but it seemed I needed to take a new direction. For a while it was all a bit confusing.

Then one day in meditation, I realized that all I had been learning, everyone I had been listening to, was talking about the same thing. I felt a great wave of love go through me. I felt I was in love with the whole world. It hit me that love was at the heart of everything. It was something that is inadequately put into words, but I had the direct experience of the reality of love, in action, and in my life.

I decided I needed even more change in my life. So I took the significant step of resigning as Deputy Principal and finally left teaching altogether.

In March 1987, a lady I was close to through the counselling work died. Two days later, the report from the latest C.A.T. scan showed my tumour still was growing. I felt — 'I have put out all this energy, done all this work, what has it been for?' For three days I stayed in bed, depressed.

During this time I really confronted the possibility of my own death. I did not eat, half meditated, half slept. I really just let go and drifted as if in another dimension for three days. My parents were really very worried about me! After three days I popped out of it. The feeling was — it was not my time to die yet: I felt as if I really had work to do. I wanted to live now — strongly! I wanted to get on with it. I went out and bought a sailing boat!

It was then as if having let go of the fear of dying, my life really began to flow. I decided to travel for a while in Canada. Then a letter from Grace arrived asking if I wanted to work for The Gawler Foundation. After a visit to Melbourne, I decided to take up the position. It felt now as if I was on my own spiritual quest, seeking my own truth, and the tumour had taken a back seat.

Before starting this new work I travelled to India and Nepal. Being in those mountains and with those people, I felt a strong sense of them being my brothers and sisters. It was in a sense a spiritual experience of feeling a oneness with people from such a different culture.

In India I visited Sai Baba and Fr. Bede Griffiths. There I met Edeltraud who has since become my wife.

It is difficult to summarize these last twelve months. It's a constant to-ing and fro-ing of understanding who I really am and feeling really very close to God. Every moment adds new learning and builds on to what I already have. It is like I am now following a direction, clear and strong in my life. At the same time it is as if there are no goals, but each moment is precious. The process is the soul part of me watching the ego part adjusting to this spiritual quality and attempting to live it day to day.

I feel a lot more humble now, and feel happy when I have this humble feeling. Working with other people is a delight, like a constant highlight. The work is putting love into practice. It is not like work for me, but a wonderful part of my life. I feel very fortunate to be able to work in this way."

Winter 1992

Frank Campbell

For Frank Campbell, cancer has led to a great deal of self knowledge and greater sense of inner peace.

It began with surgery on the back of his nose — in Melbourne, November 1984. This was followed one month later by some intravenous treatment for a tinnitus (ringing in the ears) condition. Three days later Frank noticed blood clots in his urine. He thought this must have been a consequence of the treatment, mentioned it to his doctor, but was in the process of moving to Brisbane and did not follow it up.

In Brisbane the clots came more frequently and Frank's urine became like honey. A new G.P. sent him for tests and then: "I'll never forget it, 9.20 Friday morning, I go into the doctor's surgery and he says to me — 'You look like a guy that can take it — you have a malignant cancer.' I stood up and shook his hand. 'Thank you', I said, 'I think it must have taken more guts to tell me that, than I can muster to face what I have got to.'

"I walked out of the surgery numb. I walked for two hours. As I walked I was working out what I would do with my estate. I had immediately given myself a death sentence.

"Next I was knocking on an old friend's door. She opened it and, surprised, asked me what was wrong. 'Malignant cancer,' I said. She followed with, 'Why does it always happen to the nice people.' Then she took me to my specialist urologist's examination.

"There the diagnosis was confirmed. The specialist then gave me his home phone number. 'Why do I need that?' I queried. 'You may haemorrhage over the weekend!'

"Every time I went to the toilet, I imagined I was about to bleed to death!

"On Monday, this was March 1985, by now, I had surgery to remove the malignancy. It was confirmed as an encapsulated, malignant carcinoma on a pedicle.

"After the surgery, the surgeon claimed to have successfully removed it, but was concerned about my prostate. I was booked in for more treatment in three weeks time.

"Some important things occurred while I was in hospital. When I first woke from the anaesthetic, I felt as if the lower half of my body was set on fire. Injections calmed it down. Next morning I was coming out of this reverie, when I noticed an 83-year-old gentleman opposite.

He was covered in drips and catheters and yet he was getting out of bed! 'Should you really be doing that, Old Boy.' I enquired. 'Well, no bugger's going to wipe my bum,' came the reply. 'I'm going to the toilet!'

"I looked at this guy of 83 amazed! If he can do it, why can't I. So, with some effort, I too got up and went to the toilet. It was through that man's courage at 83, the courage to do things for himself, that set me on the path to make the effort to help myself also.

"Three weeks later I was back in for the second op. The prostate was benign; it was April 1985. This time another visitor taught me a lot. He was an old friend. He called in and looking at my chart said, 'I see you're in Dr. F's weight reduction clinic.' 'I don't understand,' I replied. 'Well, I'm in too. When I get out of here I will be two stone lighter.' I then found out this man was about to have an orchiectomy (his testicles removed for prostate cancer!) This joker — on the day of his discharge after the surgery, asked his daughter to bring him in one of those bow ties with the flashing lights on them. He hid the tie in the appropriate place so that when his doctor came to examine him ...!

"Again I saw the value of a positive attitude to cancer — and humour! That gave me great inspiration.

"But now I was out and about. Unemployed, recuperating, walking 10–20km per day to build myself up, living with friends and having check-ups every three months.

"In November 1987, 14 cancer masses were discovered in my bladder wall. They were surgically removed and in December 1987, the surgeon advised me 'to begin to psychologically accept the fact that I would lose my bladder.

"At this time, I moved back to Melbourne and through a psychologist friend heard of Ian and The Gawler Foundation. That led me to do the seven day residential program which I would have to describe as the best week of my life.

"Incredible things happened to me there. I still can't explain it all. For example we did these drawings which seemed so simple. Yet they led me to learn so much about myself.

"And I had the most incredible experience. In one of the meditation sessions, touch was used by the leaders. I was lying down and first I felt a small pair of hands that seemed about 18 inches from my body. With them came a tremendous tingling and a warmth that came down over my body. The hands rested over my chest and bladder. As they left, again this sense of warmth and tingling.

"Within moments, another pair of hands, smaller, cool not hot, were felt. This time they went to my stomach and chest, then up to my forehead, back to the chest.

"Afterwards I asked David if he had touched me. He confirmed his had been the second pair. No one else had touched me! Although Eileen said that she had sent me a healing thought. I did feel healed!"

Frank was deeply moved by this experience. It had a quality and significance that had great meaning for him. A special, quite spiritual meaning.

"I come from a background in systems analysis. I still can't understand it, or understand why I was selected as if by some superior power to receive this gift. I was brought up in the Catholic Church, but somewhat rejected its dogma. With this I had the sense of a miracle coming into my life, but cannot understand why it happened, or really, accept the reality of it all.

"I went back to the hospital in March 1988. No cancer was found and since then there has been no recurrence.

"Lately, I have been completing the training program for patient contact volunteers with The Foundation. This has helped me even more. I have learnt a lot more about myself and become able to express it. In my own case, I felt that I had always been in a lockout situation.

"As a child I had a lot of stress and was unable to express it. My dad was an alcoholic and kicked me out of the house at 16 1/2. I had nothing, nowhere to go, nothing. I joined the Army, went to New Guinea, did commerce. For years I lived in other people's houses, was so busy I never had time to get to know myself.

"Finally my wife and I had our own house in Balwyn. For the first time I had a stable base, it was like a pivot point. Then the timber auction business I was in went down the tube, and with it went my marriage and house. Losing all that had a tremendous impact.

"When the cancer was first diagnosed, in a peripheral way, I thought it could have been related to the accumulated stresses. Only recently have I been able to see this relationship more rationally and objectively. I feel good about looking into all this. I feel by doing so I can become a better person — for myself — and therefore, for other people.

"I used to deeply regret those losses. Not the business so much, but the roots. I felt as if I lost my roots with the loss of marriage and house. When you go through a marriage breakup, you lose her family as well. I had a deep kinship with them. Lots of friends disappear too. I had to give away our cockatoo — it was like giving away a child — children that we never had. I had great regrets.

"What's different now? Self realization! The more one understands one's reactions to situations, the more one can be at peace with oneself. I have come to know peace within.

"I had lived in stress all my life, but did not realize it. I do now. Now I find I spend a lot more time analyzing myself. I have a lot more control. Some time ago, if someone took my space on the road I would have got really angry. Now, I just don't. I feel a lot more in control of myself. I feel a lot more responsible for myself.

"I am working long hours now. I had a long period without work. My age and health history made it hard. But now I accept that I am cancer-free. The doctors are very pleased with me and my next checkup can be done just under a local; there is no need now for the usual general anaesthetics I have had with every one in the past."

Frank found the volunteer training program has been excellent. "I came half expecting a whole lot of do gooders. You know, rich people who wanted to ease their consciences. But I found people who seriously wanted to help others; I love being with them. And I have found that if I stop long enough to listen to people, I really learn a lot. I am also learning to hear what people are really saying. This has been the greatest benefit for me in the program — learning to relate to people.

"But I also learnt a lot about myself. For years I hated my alcoholic father. He died 30 years ago and for years I carried a lot of hate and bitterness for him. I realize now that I also blamed him for lots of my own problems. It is only in these last few months, that I have been able to forgive him. It has been a great step for me and again I feel more at peace with myself. It is a joy. I feel I can speak more directly to people. I feel more content within myself. It just keeps getting better and better!"

As an extra aside, Frank is about to return to singing lessons, with a view to returning to amateur and professional work he once did. Frank also gave a talk about his experiences with cancer and The Foundation, on The Foundation's behalf, to the Rotary Club of Toorak. He is an inspiration to many and a joy to know.

October 1989

Nigel Harland

"The last lesson I learned from attending a recent residential course at Warburton was that learning to live with cancer was really just learning to live. Furthermore, that living can only be experienced in the present. I have lived an interesting life, but one which lacked purpose and direction.

"I drifted from one experience to the next. Cancer has taught me to discover myself, set my own direction and enjoy every moment of it. This requires great courage and perseverance — it may even lead to a relapse as an indication that my subconscious mind was not ready to adopt a new personality and significant stress developed in my system.

"Peace of mind exists when you act in accordance with your beliefs — I think my actions got away with me a little!

"My conclusion from this is to work harder on my beliefs. I have found great strength in that task from Anne, my partner, Karina and her wonderful support group and continual reading of Louise Hay, John Powell, Bernie Seigel and Jerry Jampolsky.

"I know I will find peace of mind, both in life and death, and my time in this life will be filled largely with joy, coupled with occasional moments of fear and frustration — these are OK for me now and I no longer try to suppress them. They pass and the joy becomes even more intense.

"Anne and I have bought a new home in Sutton Grange near Castlemaine which is a long way from the inner Melbourne suburb of Prahran where we currently live. We have left our jobs which we have worked in for a combined 35 years. We have set ourselves new and exciting goals in areas which nurture us. Our environment is utopia to us — we have everything we need. I wonder where we would be without cancer — I like it here, peace of mind, here we come!

June 1990

Annette Martin

"Two years after a mastectomy I am feeling better than I have ever felt in my life. For the first time I am at peace. No moment in the day is taken for granted. I am happy to live my life. I am aware it is a gift.

"I attended the residential program in summer 1988, six months after my operation. It took the best part of two years to recover from the shock and at the time of the residential I was still feeling fragile. I was not sure I wanted to go into a situation where I would be surrounded by people who were ill. But the experience was quite the contrary. The feeling was positive, friendly. People became very close and I experienced friendship in a way they had never known before. I shall never forget the warmth and love we shared, the inspiration and the feeling of well-being that this brought."

June 1990

Maureen Cutler

"In October 1987 I had a mastectomy and no further treatment. In October 1989 I was diagnosed as having extensive secondaries to my skull, spine, ribs and right leg. I had three weeks of radiotherapy and was put on Tamaxifen.

"In February 1990, my husband and I went to Victoria where we attended a Gawler Foundation residential cancer group. It was an intensive week of meditation, positive thinking, looking at diet and generally how to live well with a life-threatening disease.

"We returned and put it all into practice. We took up meditation, became vegetarians and my husband gave up his managerial position to work part time as a consultant and hence spend more time with me. (I gave up my job after the second diagnosis.)"

In June 1990, Maureen reported as follows:

"Saw the onco yesterday. Apparently he's a world authority on prostate and testicular cancer, so here's hoping he knows as much about bones as balls.

"A normally emotionless and extremely articulate man (it seems to go with the job), he had a lot of trouble disguising his excitement (he even looked as though he was gearing up to a hug!) and was almost reduced to a jibber on seeing my scan.

"According to him the accompanying report underestimated the 'dramatic changes' since last October. He even gave me most of the credit, as he felt the treatment was insignificant compared with my inner strength, building up an incredibly strong immune system, support etc. etc. He's in great awe of Ian Gawler and wishes his fellow colleagues, especially the older ones (he's very young) weren't so myopic."

At that time, June 1990, Maureen had recently been holidaying on Lord Howe Island where she climbed three hills; the fourth was yet to be tackled. Not bad for someone who was told she would have to give up her bushwalking!

Maureen continues:

"The dividends have paid off, as I went into remission for sixteen months. My last two bone scans in February and June have shown slight progression of the disease so I have been placed on another hormone preparation called Farlutal. I continue to keep very well, am mobile and in very little pain. I walk the dog on the beach daily, do my own gardening (I gave the housework away a long time ago!), meditate daily and go to hydrotherapy and swim nearly a kilometre twice a week.

"At the time of writing, I am planning a trip to England to stay with friends for a month. So there is life and indeed a life of quality after secondaries!"

June 1992

Doug Cowen

"I recently visited the Yarra Valley Living Centre and met Bob Sharples who asked me to put pen to paper. When he invited me to write I must admit I had the thought that it was a very unusual request. After all, what could I have to say that could be of any use or interest to others. Especially when I compare myself to Ian Gawler and the other individuals who have successfully conquered their cancer. It's been four years since I did the 'live in' course with Ian and Grace and for that four years I've been journeying along a path, literally, of life and death.

"Medically my leukemia has reached a critical stage — a stage they didn't tell me about back four years ago — then it was simply stage one, two, three, four, and you're out.

"It's not that I've come to terms with my death, and it's not that I don't want to keep on living; it's more like a realization that I've spent so much time in the past trying not to die that I forgot to live. The lessons I've learnt now, have changed my concept of living from a mere existence of plodding along, to a search for and acting out of a life of creative joy.

"I can remember reading and listening to people who carefully explained what I could/should be doing and being in utter disbelief of these buffoons — perfectly healthy people who, I thought, could have no understanding of what I was going through, what with my fears and pain and the anguish of knowing I was dying.

"I had diets, exercises, vitamins, herbs, religion, philosophy, initiations, healings, psychic readings, astrological charts, soul attunements and even got a new name. I tried being 'good', 'giving up', tried being bad and got to a point of knowing that more chemotherapy, more Christ, a different diet, more Sai Baba, a miracle herb: all seemed no different from each other.

"In fact my feeling — my inner true self — seemed to be showing me the helplessness of looking for a solution outside myself. The mysterious "turning inward" appeared to be the only path that had any substance and, ironically, the only path that offered no instant miracle solution to my health problem.

"My cancer is a relatively slow progressive type tha does not generally respond to any medical treatment. Many is the time I wished for a specific growth so that I could just take myself to surgery and get them to cut out the cancer and be done with it. However my type of disease simply forced me to take responsibility. It seems that each of us, in some weird way, gets exactly the right illness and circumstances that creates a path that is appropriate for our learning and growing.

"So what can I say to you (and really to myself)?

— two litres of cabbage juice a day will save you
— Dr. X knows of a miracle exercise
— Dolphins can show you the secret of life
— Christ heals
— four drops of selenium will do it
— love is the answer
— Vitamin C shots will eat up the cancer.

"A journey of a thousand kilometres begins with just one step" is a famous quotation. Our own path is exclusive and unique for each of us and it is always in front of us. What a joy to break free and take that first step.

"For me, I've lost count of how many steps I've taken, but along the journey I've found that I can let go of the fear and just love taking each next step.

"Although I can't see the beginning and end of my path to health while I'm walking it, I can allow myself to have faith that I've just taken the second last step. With that thought in mind I've found I've even got time to enjoy the scenery.

P.S. I think dolphins do have the secret of life. I offer a sailing trip to meet them to any of you that can make it to Byron Bay.

March 1992

Mike Nicholas

A heartwarming account of recovering from lung cancer and renewing life

"It has been a year now since my operation to remove the right lung (January 10, 1991) and many months since the course at Jumbunna. Since that time the only major medical setback was the development of a broncho-pleural fistula off my windpipe. I popped a staple. Depressingly, the top surgeons at Royal Prince Alfred and Royal North Shore Hospitals said that such a thing does not heal and would require an operation as big as that needed to remove my lung.

"On top of that, no radio or chemotherapy for the probable mediastinal metastases as too dangerous for other organs. "Yerronyerown', they said.

"Last week's C.A.T. scan showed no metastases anywhere and showed also that the broncho-pleural fistula had 'spontaneously' healed.

"My G.P. can't believe it, nor can my chest specialist. My surgeon, who said that he would take up religion if the broncho-pleural fistula healed, has been sent a Bible, two sticks of wood to make into a Cross and directions to the nearest Church to his rooms. I think he is also reviewing his betting habits.

"It would appear that I am on the way to a probable recovery. That's excessive use of the future pluperfect or subjunctive but you should be a master of it!

"I can't put my finger on any one thing that produced this result. I have no evidence that one practice is more efficacious than another. On the other hand, your records might show a pattern so I will take the liberty of telling you what my regime was in the hope that it might be useful.

1. *Meditation and Diet*

"I found it very useful to continually dip into your books, particularly *You Can Conquer Cancer.* I mean on a daily basis. It is easy to forget things, and just like it is hard changing from meat based recipes it is also hard changing lifestyle. Quite a sustained period of both constant practice and referring back to the 'service manual' is necessary, I found.

"I have been meditating for about 20 minutes daily since the course. I alternate 'white light' visualization with the 'ataraxic' meditation, i.e. the 'don't think about a white horse' one. Sometimes I mix them; beginning always with visualisation.

"Occasionally, the time varies up to one hour. I notice that after ten or twelve minutes of meditation I can see irridescent blue light.

"My feeling is that I should start putting in more work on meditation now to counteract relaxing now that the danger is over. It isn't.

"So I will enrol in an advanced course with you. Diet is vegetarian except for deep sea fish and some skinless chicken. I try to maximise vegetables that are supposed to contain selenium.

"I have gone a bit towards macrobiotics, but disagree with their view of tropical fruits. You've got to be able to look forward to a mango if the first course is brown rice, lentils and wakame seaweed! I do take some calves' or lambs' liver now and again, but try to keep protein down to about 30 gm per day.

"I've gone slack on juices. Carrot juice and barley grass or 'green magma' about twice a week. Herbal (Rener) tea once or twice daily along with Swedish bitters and a couple of swigs of chlorophyll. Stress reduction is achieved by exercise and alcohol in excessive quantities (over 40 gm/day).

"I can hear you now. 'Bump up meditation, reduce grog.' Will try.

2. *Other Treatments:*

"I'm injecting with Iscador regularly. The effects of this are supposed to be potentiated by injection also of Formica (ant juice).

"This anthroposophical regime is supposed to be illegal under the new rules. It is, of course, legal everywhere else including New Zealand!

"A friend of mine also harmonises my chakras. I meditate while she does it. I don't really understand what this is about, but I feel refreshed after the session so why complain?

"To my mind, and I hope I'm not carrying on too much, the initial surgery was vital to this recovery. I don't really think that my doctor with his 'I wish I'd never operated on you' attitude really understands even now that some cancers are very responsive to good surgery. In my case the cancer was slow growing and of the large cell type.

"This provided the time for a new dietary and meditative regime to settle in and become efficacious. I've no way of measuring the effects of the Iscador other than to say that it has to date been closely associated with a prolonged remission (horrible word!).

"All my reading has convinced me that cancer has very close nutritional associations. If we accept that it is a dynamic condition which exists in our bodies ready to go when given the right environment, then we should do our best to provide the 'hostile environment'.

"I am sure that the no fats, low protein regime does exactly that.

"As well as channelling energy into keeping the cancer at bay I am convinced that meditation had a lot to do with healing the fistula in my windpipe. While I had an 85% chance of the cancer recurring in the first year, there was absolutely no chance the fistula would heal, according to the experts.

"So I must thank you both for providing me with the means for living. It is certainly not over yet, but the odds are now in my favour."

March 1992

Nancy Daly

Nancy recently sent a long letter in reply to our follow-up questionnaire. Nancy attended a residential program in February, 1989. She noted that she first heard of the Gawler program through the cancer support group in Albury. Her local G.P. fully supported her intention to attend the program. Nancy writes in her questionnaire, "I reached my five-year mark in March. I might or might not get longer life than others on the 'orthodox trail' ... but no way would I trade my 'living' for theirs".

"My life has been tumbling over with such speed ... and fascination ... I've found it extremely difficult to 'keep up with the writing'. I'm into my 3rd volume ... and it is only the last couple of months I haven't felt such urgency to write. 'Strange' things are still happening to me, but not with such ferocious rapidity ... I seem to be 'levelling out' a bit.'

"Every facet of my life has changed, very much for the better ... and I am yet another who says that cancer is the best thing that ever happened to me. Without it, I wouldn't have learnt *any* of this, and I wouldn't have missed this experience for quids! It has not only been a learning experience for me, but for my family as well, scattered in just about every state. Their support has been tremendous ... and *my* enthusiasm has rubbed off on *them* ... and their friends ... and for a while I had an unofficial interstate postal counselling service, as letters and phone calls came from those needing support.

"Ian's 10-day self-help seminar was undoubtedly the turning point for me ... he taught us so very much, and gave us so many paths to follow ... and in my quest to 'go natural' rather than 'orthodox', I can only say 'it's been fantastic fun trying'.

"Meditation ... Oh, I am hooked! I *love* it! Especially the 'insight'. Boy! Have I learnt plenty! I'm sure I must have run the fullest gammut of meditations ... I cannot envisage what else there could be! I've seen no sign of 'evil' at all; I find the clarity incredible; I'm quite certain all our answers are within us; I've never been 'frightened', though some have been quite traumatic emotionally; and some have left me thinking 'I can do anything'. I've met two inner guides and my cartoonist sense of humour — in person ... and my guides always win their arguments — eventually! However, my guides have set me on the right track and on my own two feet, and confident I don't need them now, have left me in the hands of my 'trilogy' — my naturopath, doctor and myself. With that lot looking after me — all giving me enough rope to nearly hang myself, but not quite; all gentle, but firm when I need/ed it ... I feel I haven't got a worry in the world, healthwise.

"I've become a 'course and seminar tripper' ... continually topping-up my positivity and what I've learnt; and as I've made everyone and everything my support system ... I have so many working for my good, I wouldn't have the nerve to get sick! I now include anything that interests me — not only cancer related and include anything that interests me — not only cancer related and that is just about everything! I write all those up too — there is so much information at these, I can't see how anyone can retain any of it, without taking notes. Wherever I go — so does my folder.

"I've found there is so much more to life than I could ever have envisaged — and life now is so exciting. I simply do not know what I did for the first 57 years — it wasn't 'living' as I know it today.

"Love the newsletters, and thanks for the bit on Stephen and Edeltroud ... I often wonder how he is going. I agree with Ian on 'confidence' — your 'belief' is your key ... and Ian's program strengthened mine 'limitlessly'. It also took the fear out of cancer, and also of dying ... two very important components. Teaching, without a ruffle, dying people how to comfort other dying people ... showed superb confidence ... and I still 'giggle in awe' at the very concept ... but I wouldn't have missed it for quids either.

"One of the biggest joys of my 'learning' is about 'synchronicity' ... I'd never heard of the word — but now I literally 'live it' and love it ... I always seem to be in the right place at the right time; pick up the right book — open at the right place; meet the right people etc. etc. It happens to me all the time.

"Do you have another Sydney date for Ian yet? I know somebody interested. When he was there early May, I was at the Natural Health Autumn Convention at Stanwell Tops, and so was Avni Sali who told me he would come up to Albury and speak on 'Does Your Mind Matter' ... Boy! Does it Ever! Sometime after August he said, so our support group secretary is working on that, and we're looking forward to it very much."

June 1992

Colin Hart

"How well I remember Christmas 1987. It will be etched into my brain and I guess my family's forever. That is when I was given the diagnosis of cancer.

"I had been admitted to hospital for the removal of some polyps in the bowel. I knew there was something wrong as I woke up next morning still in hospital. It was then I was told that the doctors had found a 'thumping big tumour in the bowel, restricting it by some seven-eighths'. I had had no obvious symptoms of this condition so it came as quite a shock to me and my family.

"Surgery was scheduled for Christmas Eve 1987 and we all thought what a way to spend Christmas, but the surgeon was quite hopeful that once the tumour had been removed all would be well. However, the tumour was found to have metastasized to the outer wall of the bowel and the lymphatic system nearby. It was removed without too much of a problem, but at the same time two tumours were noticed in the liver. This was bad news.

"New Year's Day 1988, we knew the extent of the bad news. Three to six months I was told, and our world fell apart. In two weeks I had been changed from a person with the expectation of a long and healthy retirement to someone with only a few months to live. Chemotherapy was offered, but on enquiry I was told that it only had a 40% chance of holding the tumours and I would possibly have some horrible side effects. I figured that, if I only had such a short time to live, then I wanted to be as fit and well as I could for that period. I refused the offer. I believe now that that was probably a major point in my life. I was actually taking control of my life again.

"A visit from Petrea King helped me to establish some long-term goals — to be alive on my grand-daughter's 21st birthday and she was only two then. Joan, my wife, had been a community educator for the Health Department teaching cancer patients relaxation and stress management and how to cope with their cancer for some years, and knew what complementary help was available. She had also been interested in the work of Ian and Grace Gawler for many years.

"I decided to try their approach and attended the Gawlers' residential program as soon as I was well enough. The second major decision had now been made and as it turned out, was to be probably the most significant factor in my recovery. I wasn't looking forward to being with a lot of sick people (that's what cancer had conjured up in my mind) so I was pleasantly surprised to find that few of the participants were really sick. I was plunged into a world I had never experienced before. Meditation, positive attitudes, diet, secrets of drawings (wow! that was an eye-opener), positive thinking, power of the mind, beliefs and how they work on you, affirmations, attitudinal healing, peace of mind, communication skills, and many more. There were sad moments too. I can remember being able to judge what sort of session we were in for by the number of boxes of tissues distributed around the room.

"It was at this residential program that I 'got the message'. It was during a hands on healing meditation that I had a very powerful experience which really 'blew my mind'.

"I had an overwhelming feeling of peace and calm and from that moment on, felt that all my worries, anxieties and fears left me and I was at peace with the world. Even as I write these words the feeling has come back as it always does when I tell my story to others. It is a truly wonderful feeling. It left me walking on air for the rest of the residential.

"As I was telling Joan about this experience, I had almost an uncontrollable urge to do something for other cancer patients. I didn't know what form it would take, but Ian was offering his first leaders' training program three weeks later, so we arranged with him to come back to do this course. It was interesting to go through what we learnt during the residential program from the other side, i.e. learning how to teach those things. Having cancer, I believe, was a great help here.

"It was always Joan's ambition to start a support group in our area for cancer patients and their carers so we made the decision to start as soon as we could.

"With the doctor's predictions in the back of our minds, we cautiously began to rebuild our lives. One thing we did was to take an around-the-world trip nine months after diagnosis for three and a half months. So much for predictions. As time passed we noticed that the tumours, whilst not gone, were only growing at a slow rate, so I embarked on a process of learning more about stress management and relaxation and what could be done by patients for themselves. I became more and more convinced that the key lay in keeping the immune system functioning at its maximum capacity and in the power of positive thinking.

"This was a really fascinating area to explore. Prior to diagnosis I had worked all my life as an accountant. As I experimented with the use of affirmations and noticed the changes taking place within me, I was convinced that the manner in which I had been brought up, trained, and influenced by all sorts of things, were all presenting a negative attitude, so I had become a very negative person. Please do not think that I had a horrible childhood etc. Far from it, but the influences on me were no different from those to which the bulk of the population were subject. These attitudes have been handed down from generation to generation and it's only now, at 62 years of age, I am starting to see how destructive negative 'self talk' can be if not corrected.

"Another area which I explored was the connection between the mind and how you felt. Mind you I am no psychologist and all I could go on was my observations. I noticed that as I became more positive, so I felt better. Scientists have known for some time about the stress response and I was able to see how this affected me. If I was tense then I felt poorly, and so I reasoned that, if we do produce chemicals which suppress the immune system, as we are told, and I could observe it in myself, then it was logical that the opposite could be put to good use in keeping me well.

"I also observed in our groups that when we talked about positive thinking and the effect of all that negative 'self talk' we had absorbed and then put into practice some simple affirmation like 'I am a positive person now' the change in them was almost immediate. Their posture improved, their voice tones changed into much stronger positive notes, their faces became alive, and they felt good, sometimes for the first time since diagnosis.

"I get a great buzz out of seeing these changes take place, because I know what it is like, I've been there and experienced it all.

"My tumours continued to grow slowly, and surgery for their removal was offered. This involved an operation to remove part of the liver. At that time I wasn't keen to have the operation as I considered the odds, so surgery was deferred.

"Surgery was again suggested three years after diagnosis and once again I refused it as I didn't feel right about it. I guess that I wasn't sure if I had any further tumours in my body. I had seen two friends die within seven months after such surgery as a result of further tumours becoming apparent.

"However, last October, I explored the option of surgery again. The tumours were just starting to make their presence felt, although I was well and doing all those things I had always done, like playing tennis and golf. A complete check of my body was done to see if any other tumours were apparent. After some four years none were observed, so I decided that the time had come to be rid of the two I still had. Surgery was performed in December 1991 and involved the removal of the right lobe of my liver. I must admit I wasn't very well for a few days after it, but as time progressed so my health improved. I was back playing tennis 10 weeks after the operation. Subsequent tests have shown that I have no tumour activity in my body and my liver has regrown.

"I guess I have been fortunate to have been married to my 'support group' as Joan has been of enormous help in managing to meet my dietary requirements over the last four years and been there when I had a problem with visualization and when disappointments arose following C.A.T. scans which didn't show the results we were both looking for. Only now has she expressed her opinions as to my decisions not to have surgery in the early years and I thank her for standing by me and letting me make those decisions myself. It must have been very hard to stand back at that time and say nothing. Her help has gone a long way in helping me achieve what I have.

"Where do I go from here? My guess is that I will continue my work with cancer patients, but one thing for sure is that I cannot become complacent. Meditation, positive attitudes and a healthy diet have become so much a part of my life now, that I will continue the practice in the future.

"Just the simple knowledge that what I am doing for myself is right for me, is probably the basis on how I live now. I've done my research, made my decisions and am now getting on and living to the best of my ability for as long as I have got, with no fear for the future."

October 1992

Joyce Oag

Cancer has been my teacher and I have been a slow learner. But what I have learnt is that there is so much help out there to tap into if you are prepared to reach out. Simply try each path which opens up to you until you find the right one for you, i.e. the ones that touch you deeply.

I had the first malignant carcinoma in my right breast in 1986. After a radical mastectomy my lymph glands were clear and it had been analysed as a primary cancer. My surgeon felt he had "got it all" and the prognosis was very good indeed. I recovered well and got back into all the "busy-ness" of life again, feeling I had been "lucky".

Exactly two years later in 1988 I had visited my surgeon for my checkup and he was surprised to find another lump in the remaining breast. He arranged a mammogram and an ultrasound there and then, and as he had just had a patient cancel an operation the following morning, he offered to slot me into that time if I would like to take it. So after a phone call to my husband I proceeded straight to the hospital. My husband was shocked, duly arrived and agreed it was better to get it over without delay.

My surgeon followed the same procedure as the first time, i.e. removing the lump and having pathology on it whilst I was anaesthetised, and, as it was malignant, removing the whole breast and lymph glands. It was another primary cancer and oestrogen positive, whereas the first one was progesterone positive, but again my lymph glands were clear and so I felt incredibly lucky as he had "got it all". My surgeon and I both said it can't happen again. It was true enough with the loss of both breasts and very much a Pollyanna attitude.

I decided as I went to acquire my second prosthesis I now could be flexible and I chose to come down a size in bust measurement. It took me longer to recover the second time and I had to have my large Keloid scar cut and redone as it was painful and waking me at night. I had six radiation treatments to slow down the healing of the scar and I eventually started to feel comfortable once more.

I acquired Ian Gawler's books and Petra King's *Quest for Life* and read them, and so had quite an awareness now about cancer. I began making changes in my life (I slowed down somewhat), resigned from committees that I had loved being a part of and gave up doing Meals-on-Wheels. I have practised yoga for almost 20 years so I know about relaxation and meditation etc, but somehow had not honed in on it. I kept my yoga going and some more gentle things that were not so demanding and freed myself of being responsible for all sorts of rosters etc.

Then in May 1991 my world fell apart and was shattered with the result of the bone scan I had because of pain in my left ribs. The original pain was a red herring and not related to bone cancer. But it fortunately enabled early detection of the twelve secondary tumours peppered throughout my bones in the neck, spine, clavicle, arm, ribs, hips and leg. The medical treatment prescribed was Nolvadex-D (Tamoxifen) a hormone treatment taken orally.

I must say at this point I consider myself fortunate in having the wonderful doctors I have. My wonderful GP over 20 years gave me acupuncture and encouragement. Likewise my surgeon of over 15 years, whom I have the utmost faith in, helped and encouraged me. So, knowing I had the best medical help available, I knew that I must reach out and tap into the best of self-help programs that spoke to me.

What an experience and journey lay ahead. I had no idea that it could be so rewarding, fulfilling and exciting. At that point I decided that I was a very inhospitable host to this cancer invading my body and life, but as I was rapidly running out of options, decided to give it my undivided attention. Michelle (my daughter) came with me, and another wonderful friend Joan, to Ian Gawler's Sydney seminar and then we had an appointment with Petra King. I started taking juices (carrot, celery and beetroot) and supplements of Vitamins C and B to strengthen the immune system. A radical change of diet was commenced. We had learnt that if the immune system could be free of coping with chemicals, i.e. preservatives and artificial substances, caffeine and tannin etc., it could get on with the job of healing which it is good at. Michelle emptied out the pantry cupboard so I would not be tempted to use up all the refined products that sat there. Michelle stayed for a month and helped us make the changes in our die so we had everything pure and natural. She taught my wonderful husband to cook vegetable stir-fries and vegetable lasagna, etc. This was a huge change from our meat and vegies each night. The other very important ingredient is our attitude, i.e. we always prepare with love and eat with joy.

I knew at Ian Gawler's seminar we were only touching the tip of the iceberg and that I needed to do the residential program at The Yarra Valley Living Centre. My husband came down with me as my support person and we had an amazingly powerful week which changed our life for the better. We set out to remove stress from our life by working through many and various issues. I believe stress was in fact a core cause of my cancer and we came home with a solution. We both meditate together each morning, have a healthy pure diet and I do visualisations regularly and see myself getting rid of the cancer. We each have our own affirmations and with our positive attitude we know they work. We do more regular exercise — swimming and walking. We also learnt to set realistic goals — short term, mid and long term. The first goal being to be able to drive to Mildura in that September for the birth of our grandchild. I was in fact well enough to do that and be there for our granddaughter's arrival and also to be of help. I attended wool embroidery classes and made our precious new granddaughter a beautiful embroidered baby blanket. It gave me so much joy doing this wonderful creative work. I continue with my yoga and find that it is an important part of my week.

I have had regular visits to my very good and supportive oncologist and each quarterly scan showed gradual improvements, with some tumours diminishing in size. I always ask to see my scans so I can know exactly where they (the tumours) are so whilst visualising I could go right to the very spot.

However, I was still lacking in energy, e.g. I would sleep for 12 hours and still be tired and sleep each afternoon. I kept being led to reiki and I witnessed what it did for another cancer patient at Yarra Valley and decided I would like to do the reiki Seminar in August 1992. My friends and acquaintances could not stop telling me how well I looked and I then completed reiki II in December. What pleased me about reiki was that as well as being able to do it for others I was able to do it for myself. Simply hands on and no matter how tired I was feeling, and no matter where I was, I could always put my hands on and feel that universal life force. I have more energy and vitality now than even before cancer.

I then had my December scan and it was all clear of any active cancer. Truly a miracle. So now there is no way we change our lifestyle as it is far better than life before cancer. The whole experience has taught us how very precious life is and never to take it for granted. We live in the moment and enjoy each day.

Love is the key and I have so much surrounding me from my family and wonderful friends. Our son cut short his overseas holiday to be with us to help and his help was so valuable in pointing us in the right direction. My wonderful friend, Yvonne (we have been friends since age seven) was a constant tower of strength and understanding, loving support. I could go on all day naming friends, they know who they are and how important they have been in my life.

My wonderful husband has always remained positive and we share so much more than ever before.

I believe that another important part of my healing is that I have learnt to say *no*.

So ... I continue to set more realistic goals and look forward to the next half of my life with hope and joy. I no longer am afraid of cancer. I am certainly more in touch with my higher self and higher power. I have a peace of mind now that is a priceless gift and my heart is full of gratitude.

August 1993

Quentin Blayney (1974–1993) by his mother

Quentin's first brain tumour symptoms occurred on Christmas Day 1985, when he was eleven years and ten months of age. He underwent neurosurgery, which resulted in a left sided paralysis. He was forced to change from right to left hand dominance. Extensive radiotherapy followed, resulting in retarded spinal growth. It was during this time that we contacted The Gawler Foundation (then ACPF), to help Quentin to embrace a positive approach to his condition. He spent the time talking and drawing with Ian, completing a remarkable series of drawings with his left hand.

Following a remission the cancer relapsed and after further surgery in 1989, Quentin returned to The Foundation to learn to meditate. He then accompanied me on a brief trip abroad to visit the major galleries in New York, Paris and London, and to see old friends. (I had been told he was unlikely to live beyond six months.) The tumour recurred in 1990 and surgery then resulted in severe hemiplegia, a permanent limp and useless right arm.

Quentin was undaunted and continued to pursue his life and art. After these three tumours Quentin held a successful One Man Exhibition of 27 works and won the City of Heidelberg Young Artist's Scholarship, for artists up to 25 years of age. He was sixteen years and ten months.

Early in 1991 the tumour was back, but no longer operable. Quentin focussed upon his meditation and his art and in February we attended a Residential Program at The Foundation, to reinforce the approach we were taking. Quentin then increased his meditation to three hours daily.

By the end of April he was totally blind, although sometimes hallucinating and imagining he saw things, partly due to his strong visual memory. In the months ahead he took up Blues Harmonica as a creative outlet and early the following year turned his attention to Sculpture and studying VCE English. By now part of the brain tumour had forced itself through the scarline and was growing outside the skull, and required daily nursing care. Eventually this external mass was irradiated and when it began haemorrhaging afterwards, neurosurgery was again required, to shave it back to the scalp. From this time on

Quentin needed morphine, along with his meditation practice and other drugs.

His survival and his remarkable zest for life, optimism and artistic output continued to amaze his doctors and all around him. In October 1992 he held an exhibition of 16 sculptures (as part of schools VCE art show) completed during the previous six months. Most sold and patrons requested second editions. Another operation was required to again debulk the external tumour in November. He passed VCE English and continued to sculpt and play harmonica.

By early 1993, there was a metastases in a neck lymph node as well. Quentin won the Tattersall's Award for Enterprise and Achievement for his exceptional creativity and the example he set others. He died on April 24th 1993 — aged nineteen years and nine weeks.

At his funeral, Ian spoke and quoted the artist Paul Gaughin, "Life is hardly more than a fraction of a second; such a little time to prepare oneself for eternity". Quentin left so very well prepared.

Caring for Quentin: A Teenager with Cancer, by Paula deBurgh

When Quentin's cancer first appeared, I had already been divorced for four years and my former spouse had moved interstate. Thus I was to become the primary care giver and sole parent throughout the illness with occasional brief visits from Quentin's father. My life was the only one that was radically adjusted by the cancer, apart from Quentin's, and our experience probably matches those of others in our predicament. The period of time for Quentin's first symptoms until his death was seven years and four months.

It took a year to deal with all the exigencies of Quentin's first brain tumour and for life to return to some semblance of normality, and for me to get back to my professional life. Soon after the relapse in 1989 with its pessimistic prognosis for Quentin's survival I sometimes wondered if and when I would be able to retrieve my own life. After the next year in a state of suspended animation, (caring for Quentin through his operations and rehabilitation and knowing he could die at any time) I decided to place my personal life aspirations on the back burner, and focus upon each day as it unfolded. Having made this choice, I found that I attained peace of mind and could give myself whole-heartedly to Quentin's struggle. (Later I wrote at night for some mind space, but it wasn't my primary focus).

I sensed it was important that Quentin retain his individuality and autonomy — by deciding what activities he wished to pursue; what clothing, diet, study or social life he desired, when he would meditate and so on. I discovered very early that it was essential not to discourage new interests and activities just because a person may be terminally ill. In fact Quentin's most outstanding achievements occurred in the four years after the relapse of his cancer — but even if he had not soared so high, the activities would have been worthwhile in their own right. Quentin held a vision of the future, which I encouraged, and this sustained him through what, on one level were the horrific trials of his illness. He used art, then music, then sculpture and study to challenge the despair of his potentially short life.

As Quentin's various functions became impaired and his independence compromised, I saw myself as the facilitator for his quality of life, and ensured that the materials or resources he required to continue to express his individuality were available to him. I realised that a carer is not valued within society and there is nothing tangible to show for the years of love and effort one invests. There are no rewards in death, except the knowledge that you did all that was humanly possible to enhance the life of your charge.

After Quentin's third operation in 1990, he was abandoned by most of his peer group. This was a source of great distress to him, while he understood that it was the fear that he would die that had driven them away. To partly compensate for this loss and to help lift his spirits we adopted a little dog, which he named Flynn. His animal was a great joy to him until the end and is now in my care. Eventually, some of his friends returned.

When there was an obvious shift in his condition (e.g. the onset of blindness; appearance of an external tumour), Quentin would be touchy and bloody-minded with me for days, until we uncovered the source of his anxiety, which was generally, "that I'm getting worse". He called this treatment of me "cruel love", as a teenager will only pick on the person they feel safest with. In the last year of his illness this no longer occurred, as we'd short-circuit the situation and laugh instead.

With an adolescent, issues of emerging sexuality and identity crop up, along with the realisation that if the illness progresses, they will probably never have a partner. I had to tackle this with Quentin and through the assistance of a male friend his needs were provided for.

As a sole carer, I lacked the emotional support that couples can offer one another when a child is ill. Thus I wore two hats. As well as being comforter, nurse, carer and person who adapted to the unpredictability of Quentin's symptoms, I was also organiser, administrator and person who liaised with doctors, nurses, relatives and friends. Sometimes the fatigue level was unimaginable, as I could only engage a council carer for five hours a week due to limited funds. Other time off depended upon the goodwill of siblings and friends — and such goodwill tended to diminish as the years passed.

In this state of chronic tiredness, I pre-arranged Quentin's funeral — which at the time was the most odd and difficult experience of my life — especially as I hoped he would survive ... Later I was glad I had, as on the day following his death, I was in no fit state to do so. For the last two years of Quentin's life, he knew he was not likely to win and we spoke openly about the possibility of death — although one had to be judicious in choosing the right moment. I found that approaching the matter obliquely worked best, such as: "If we don't win this fight dear, is there anything particular you feel you need to say? ... What would you like done with your ashes? ... Any particular way you'd like to be remembered", etc. etc. By the time Quentin died, we'd discussed his anxieties, wept about the possibility of him dying, aired his fears, handled resolvable conflicts with others and ensured there was no unfinished business. And then he kept living as fully as possible.

November 1993

Ray Hasegawa

It has been 12 months since my operation for bowel cancer. On 18th May I was diagnosed with metastatic tumours on both lobes of my liver; some weeks later I attended the 23rd June 1991 residential.

Your programme confirmed many of my own beliefs and taught me the skills of meditation. On returning home I attended the Peter McCallum Cancer Institute, where they offered me chemotherapy. I took some weeks researching the drugs they offered me and on the fourth week I told them I would not have the chemotherapy.

My oncologist was very supportive and offered a system based on blood tests and physical examinations to monitor my progress. I was happy with this and returned home to put all my knowledge into practice. I adopted a very strong, positive thinking attitude, P.M.R., and imagery meditation, the maintenance diet and exercise. Within six months I had visited the Peter McCallum about six times. Each visit showed remarkable progress in that I gained weight and was not showing any of the symptoms that the oncologist questioned me about.

Early this year (1992) my original oncologist went on confinement leave, so I now have another oncologist, my visits went from once a month to every six weeks and, for 1992, are now every eight weeks. My last visit on 29th April, to my surprise, the oncologist called me the miracle case and remarked that if it was not for my file no one would believe I had cancer. He then for the first time showed interest in what I was doing. I walked out of there very pleased and with a smile on my face that was infectious because, as I walked the streets of Melbourne, I noticed people were smiling at me. I felt great!

Here is a list of my personal beliefs that I live by:

- A very strong positive attitude (which has not wavered).
- Meditation (P.M.R. and imagery).
- Diet (Maintenance).
- Exercise: I walk every day, play golf approx. three times a week, play tennis once a week, bike ride, and snow ski approximately 20 days every winter. Must mention 1991: three months after my operation I was skiing on Mt. Hotham and, to my surprise, outskiing my friends.

- Stress control: I have retired and changed my lifestyle.
- Live alone: As I do live alone, I am not in conflict; this gives me space and time to look after myself. No-one to seek approval from; no-one to make demands. I live my life alone, but I am not lonely.
- Support: I have wonderful support from my children, family and friends.
- Quality of life: Since the day my doctor told me I have cancer, the quality of my life has made a quantum leap.
- Responsibility to oneself (to take control of one's own life).

The above list is my everyday experience and will be for life.

It has come to me that I have not mentioned being drug free. Even before my diagnosis I had not been on any medication; this I mean for 57 years. I have never even experienced a headache, so no analgesics. Five days before leaving hospital I refused medication, and to this day have not had any medication. All my life I have had a belief that the body heals itself psychologically and physically.

I wish to be reminded to all those who shared the June 1991 residential, and to all cancer patients and others who seek to take control of their own lives and live with inner peace and be in harmony with the universe.

February 1993

Wensley Roth

Wensley was diagnosed with non-Hodgkins lymphoma in November 1990. She had several enlarged lymph nodes removed from her upper arm, but then no other treatment. She is in full remission and living a joyous life. Her story focuses on finding the spiritual meaning in her disease and life, and how, for her, this has been, and remains, the way to her ongoing health and wellbeing.

"On the last visit to my oncologist in July I was told 23% of patients with the type of lymphoma that affected me have spontaneous remission. This being the result of how the patient treats their body, their mental attitude and the healing methods used. The methods one patient uses do not necessarily help another. This suggests to me that spontaneous remission occurs not only as a result of a process of mind, but an intangible state of being beyond the mind, varying in degree or intensity in each individual, immeasurable and unpredictable because the outcome of all preparation and effort depends on the individual and the grace of God.

I believe by the practise of meditation we create the right conditions to receive divine grace, preparing our mind and body for this wonderful gift by expressing love.

When we concentrate on love of God, love of inner self, love of self, love of humanity, love of nature, then God will confirm WE ARE LOVE.

The affirmations I worked on during the residential program are as follows:

At last I can be my 'true self' I realise this body is mortal and I have much to achieve in this incarnation.

Spiritual evolvement is the number-one priority in my life. All that matters is *love* and I feel free to express it.

For a short time I added 'aspiring' to immortality because the affirmation said 'I am immortal'. I had in mind a Baba prayer, part of which says 'Lead me from mortality to immortality' meaning liberation. I remember the whole class agreed that we do not give enough consideration to the fact that we may die earlier than one expects. We must realise we do not live on earth forever and must use our time here wisely. By saying 'my body' is mortal takes care of the soul aspect — rather than saying, 'I am mortal'.

During a period in my life years previously when I practised yoga and meditation I was given by the grace of God, the spiritual experience of Unification. In a state of heightened awareness and transcendence I found my soul's true identity and relationship to God and the universe. Actually there is no relationship or duality at the highest; all is one. I rarely spoke of this knowledge, never asserting myself in this direction.

I was shown I was here on earth to learn, but my spiritual goal of overcoming the emotions and ego, evolving into a higher being, was becoming more remote as a result of my lifestyle; family and career being my priorities. My spiritual life was existing in slow motion and I was always conscious of an unfulfilled yearning within.

It took a hard lesson like being confronted with disease to give impetus to my spirituality and a return to meditation practice.

These positive attitudes contributed towards my return to health. I hope they can be of assistance in helping others along the path. Listen to your inner voice. To have approval of one-self is more important than looking to others for approval.

Attend to your needs without consciously hurting others. I learnt during the program that we cannot go through life always putting other peoples' needs and feelings before our own. This can lead to emotions of frustration, resentment, guilt and anxiety depleting the immune system by stress etc.

If someone should be hurt as a result of my action that is entirely their reaction over which I have no control. Then I must ask, 'What is the lesson in this for me?' Maybe another time I could take a different approach or attitude.

Follow your path of spiritual evolvement for a healthy mind and sound body. The ideal is to allow yourself freedom of expression directed towards the highest principles endeavouring to guide thoughts, words and actions with love.

It is essential that body and mind, thoughts, words and actions make a harmonious whole to gain equanimity and health. I try to live in the present without worrying about the past, try not to think ahead such as being engaged in doing one thing and already thinking about the next task. To make a list of tasks to be done concentrating fully on each separately avoids anxiety.

Because of the illumination I received through meditation I am able to avoid the negative energy of the fear of death which detracts from one's well being and which is enervating to one who is ill. Death is a natural part of life and I know that when the time comes for my death it will be a beautiful experience. I will be taken up by an outpouring of divine splendour and love to merge with the absolute.

Each one of us is a divine being sustained by God. I now strive to live in the constant awareness of this truth.

In the past I woke up with a feeling of peace which was quickly overshadowed by a feeling of apprehension as I became fully awake.

Since my change of attitude to acknowledge my inner self and divinity once again, to love God with more intensity, to be receptive to His love, I wake with a warm feeling of contentment, love and peacefulness that is carried into my waking state and which I try to keep or recapture during the day. I find it again during meditation and I believe with practice this inner peace will be of longer duration.

I was given an insight that the object of the disease was to bring me to Sai Baba. The law of synchronicity became apparent in my life when I attended your residential program; being introduced to Baba's vibhutti and buying the book by Sam Sandweiss when we lunched at the administration. It was not a coincidence that I met some Baba devotees shortly after.

Time after time Baba confirms to me what I have experienced as truth through his sayings, discourses, and dreams."

February 1995

Sue Dixon

Cancer! I sat there in disbelief as the surgeon proceeded to tell me that I had carcinoma of the breast and would need a mastectomy. I'd always imagined I'd die of heart disease which seemed to run in the family — not cancer. I'd breast-fed my three children for years, been meditating for years and ate what I thought was a healthy diet. I felt cheated and incredibly scared. It would take some time before I could begin to understand all the factors that contributed to me getting cancer.

July 1990: Mastectomy. Return to four day per week work as a family therapist, working with children and families in violent and sexually abusive situations, five weeks later. This was a week after my husband had an emergency appendectomy. One month later he had a breakdown and would not return to full-time work for six months. We were struggling in our 22-year-old marriage. So I took up full-time work and the following year took steps to start my masters degree. I kept wondering if I had made enough changes to prevent getting secondaries, but I had made myself too busy to think too much.

May 1992: Large mass (4cm x 8cm) discovered in the right lobe of my liver and 2cm ones scattered throughout the left lobe. I felt utterly devastated, full of self-blame for not making the necessary changes, full of guilt for the children's sakes and very angry. The doctors basically wrote me off, saying there was a very small chance tamoxofin would help (it isn't very effective in pre-menopausal women) and I reluctantly decided to go on it. I re-read *You Can Conquer Cancer* and began to piece together an understanding of why I'd got cancer in the first place and why I'd got secondaries. So many factors including my perfectionist nature, living my life according to others expectations, pleasing behaviours, first child—highly responsible, believing it was up to me to make people feel better … and so on.

It felt like months of misery combined with a sense of panic that I did not have the positive attitude I needed to heal myself. But I was also aware that for the first time I was allowing myself to feel negative emotions instead of burying them and denying them as I'd always done, out of fear.

And then with the help of Ysha, my wonderful acupuncturist, I began to feel brave enough to face the issue of marriage. I began to realise that I was more fearful of leaving it than I was of dying and that somehow I'd given myself a death-wish because I felt there was no way out of this long, long and unhappy relationship. I was faced with the fact that relative comfort and convenience and keeping up appearances had kept me there. If, as Pema Chodron said in *The Wisdom of No Escape*, one has the courage to face inconvenience and uncertainty, one can slowly but surely transform one's way of thinking, one's life.

To help me make the move I decided to do a 10-day residential course at The Gawler Foundation. This was a wonderful experience and it gave me the strength and wisdom to go home and end the relationship. There I also faced my great reluctance to work really hard at this healing business, to be a 100 percenter! I now see how very difficult it is to begin to turn around one's deep-seated beliefs about unworthiness and self-blame, to even begin the work effectively. But one has to start somewhere and I felt so inspired by meeting Ian and knowing others who had healed themselves. I also had wonderful support from my dear friend Trish who has stood by me through everything. Also my faith in my Tibetan Buddhist teachers and my meditation practices.

I began to feel that for the first time since beginning meditation in 1982, I knew how to meditate, to stop 'doing' meditation and simply sit in mindfulness with no attachment to outcome. I felt that my visualisations were very powerful—white light washing over my liver, washing away my cancer cells, then golden light washing over my completely healthy liver. I couldn't visualise it being clear of cancer until I stopped believing I deserved to get sick.

January 1993: Facing death, moving past the denial (oh, it is so painful to face one's negativities) when faced with my terrible prognosis—30% live two years, 5% live five years and 1% live 10 years. Sogyal Rinpoche's book *The Tibetan Book of Living and Dying* helped me prepare a daily death preparation practice which I find invaluable. And I have no fear of death now.

April 1993: Follow-up course at The Gawler Foundation. Once again more profound changes as after talking to my other wonderful support person, Bob Sharples, I realised that I could not return to part-time work and study as I'd planned to. Whilst I felt well, I still needed to learn how to break the busy pattern and learn to be still and quiet. Very traumatic as I faced my deep attachment to my identity as a therapist/senior team member/public servant. If I wasn't those things, who was I?

May 1993: Investigations showed no tumours left in my liver! I was elated and had a party to thank all my friends, and my poor parents who'd been so distressed, for all their prayers and support. So many of their friends and relatives had prayed for my recovery.

And so I became a 100 percenter. Meditating for three hours a day, keeping to the maintenance diet strictly, having five to six juices a day, vitamin supplements, exercising, etc. 1993 was a very tough year as my daughter struggled with the separation and her fears about me dying, in her final year at school. I see now how much I tried to protect them and not let them know how distressed I was feeling so much of the time, and how guilty I felt for getting sick. I'd do it differently now. Kids shouldn't be protected. They know anyway. Tough year too as I adjusted to living alone after 24 years, being a single parent, having no money, selling the family house, being like my clients on a disability pension, having no real sense of who I was after all the years of living according to others' expectations. I began to accept that obstacles are part of life and they are a major opportunity for growth and transformation.

So here I am writing this a few weeks off two years after the diagnosis of the secondaries and I'm clearly a 100 percenter. I'm working now in private practice after making the enormous decision to leave the public service, knowing that I have to follow my heart. I'm teaching meditation and counselling a few people, some with cancer, and running an "Enhancing Your Health" group for women. I've also established an exciting connection with the Vietnamese Buddhist community in South Australia (one temple in Melbourne) after a monk in Vietnam translated an article I wrote about my healing in an international Buddhist magazine and several people wrote to me in Vietnamese. Through the translator I talked to the community in South Australia and they asked me to go to Vietnam this year (1994) to see the women and the monk.

So the challenge remains—to change old patterns and beliefs, keep up two hours of meditation a day, stay on the maintenance diet pretty rigorously. I am also embarking on a thorough self-examination process using Caroline Myss and Norman Shealley's book *The Creation of Health* kindly lent to me by Grace. The path of transformation seems to involve a shedding of layer after layer of beliefs and attitudes that have propped one up all one's life. It's no wonder that (in their terms) I'm experiencing such soul-pain!

It's been really healing for me to write this because it's the first time that I've really acknowledged what I've done.

February 1995

Kevan Johnston

Dear Ian,

I hope this letter finds you well. Early February I attended the Prince of Wales Oncology Department for a check up, which was exactly 12 months to the day that my diagnosis was made. You may recall that during the October five-day live-in, we discussed my earlier report from the Prince of Wales and you asked me to place it in the file at The Gawler Foundation. I have enclosed a copy of my report for the recent visit, which you may like to read and also place in my file.

It was only at this February visit that I made them aware of my contact with The Gawler Foundation. Very early in my treatment I asked that they monitor my progress with regular blood tests. Their comment, "We won't learn anything from doing that". So, rather than argue when they were not keen, I had my local G.P. in Sydney, Dr. Stone, do the tests. This made me realise that it would be better if I did not confide in them with any alternate treatment I may decide to choose until I had the runs on the board.

I approached the February visit full of confidence and feeling well and decided to tell them what I had been doing. Dr. Michael Back, a young, enthusiastic oncologist was full of support and encouraged me to continue with the program. Unfortunately, I cannot say the same about others involved.

It is interesting to note in the report that Dr. Michael Back refers to The Gawler Foundation. I think we are winning on two fronts—my healing progress and recognition of The Gawler Foundation.

I realise that I am far from being out of the woods, but I will succeed in regaining perfect health. I continue with my daily routine of walking 9km down to the beach, where I do my breathing exercises, and back before breakfast. I am fanatical about my diet, meditation, vitamins and attitude toward life. Mid-afternoon I return to the beach with my dog Max, and walk mid-shin deep in the water for as long as I can, depending on the tide. This averages in distance about 5–6km.

Throughout the day I continue to do the many jobs around the property, without any discomfort. I plan each day to be extremely tired by the time I retire to bed. I sleep well and I have not spent any time at all dwelling on my situation.

I have had wonderful support from the leader of my medical team, Dr. Peter Blaxland, a Macquarie Street surgeon and friend of 20 years, who I have confided in and who has guided me to the best medical facilities available. I am sure I have had the best medical treatment available, although only palliative. With the enormous help from The Gawler Foundation in setting my life plan into action, I will succeed.

Since the finish of the radiation treatment in April 1993, we have lived in North Queensland where there is no pollution or stress. I have had wonderful support from a local GP, Dr. John Parker, who, after contacting Dr. Ian Brighthope, planned my intravenous vitamin C program and I was blessed to have met a wonderful naturopath, Elizabeth Bally, who has a clinic in the Coral Seas Resort, Airlie Beach. Elizabeth has an exceptional knowledge on the problems of cancer and self-healing programs, having worked with the Hoxsey Clinic. She healed her husband of cancer with no medical treatment some 10 years ago. Elizabeth will attend a support persons program at The Gawler Foundation when this can be arranged. Both Dr. John Parker and Elizabeth Bally have supported the start of the Whitsunday Cancer Support Group, with Elizabeth arranging the program for the meetings. At last Monday's meeting 23 members attended.

Ian, this may sound a little strange but I consider my cancer to be a good experience. It has changed my life. I am now leading a peaceful, non-stressed life-style with a wonderful satisfaction in my healing progress and support group.

Please ask Marion to book both Gloria and I into a five-day live-in later in the year. I look forward to seeing you again.

P.S. I have also started jogging again during my walks, preparing for the local Mini Marathon later in the year.

February 1995

Kate McMartin

I was diagnosed with medullary cell carcinoma of the thyroid in July 1991. I was 33 years old. My doctor was very encouraging and said that if you had to get cancer, mine was a particularly good one to get as it was easily treated. I was scheduled to have a total thyroidectomy in August. I was assured that it would be a simple procedure with very little side effects and a quick recovery.

When I awoke from the surgery, the story was a little different. The cancer had already spread to the lymph nodes and the surgeon had been unable to remove them all. The nodes in my chest were also affected. I was told that I would require a thoracotomy five weeks later. Radiation had been ruled out as my cancer was particularly rare and did not respond to radiation or chemotherapy. My 'particularly good cancer' was getting out of control.

The thoracotomy was considered to be fairly successful, although there was some disagreement as to whether they had "got it all".

I recovered slowly from the surgery and resumed a fairly normal lifestyle. I felt that I had been "lucky" but I did not make plans that were too far into the future. I felt like I was walking along a tightrope and could fall off at any time.

My first recurrence was diagnosed in July 1992. I had a lump half way up the side of my neck. I started a new round of tests and decided to seek out other opinions. The prognosis was very poor. I could undergo a radical dissection of both sides of my neck; that would involve removing all the lymph nodes and most of the muscles from the sides of my neck. I was told that this surgery would not cure me but I should live until I was 40! If I chose not to have the surgery I would not have very long to live.

I chose not to have the surgery. I decided that quality of life was more important to me than quantity. It was time for me to start doing something for myself. I could no longer leave it all up to someone else.

I decided to go to the Gerson Clinic in Mexico. I arrived in Tijhuana a week later with my close friend Cheryl. She had come along to support me while I was on the therapy. The Gerson therapy is a particularly rigorous diet regime which involves drinking 13 vegetable juices (mainly carrot) each day, taking a multitude of supplements to aid digestion and speed up the body's metabolism, and five coffee enemas daily (every four hours).

We stayed in Mexico for nearly a month so that I would be well and truly settled into the therapy before attempting the long trip home. One of the side effects of the Gerson therapy is 'flare-ups', which can occur once every four days to once every two weeks. The symptoms can vary from flu-like symptoms to vomiting and diarrhoea and can last two to three days. I, unfortunately, experienced a 'flare-up' every five days and these episodes left me particularly weak and delayed our departure for Australia at one point.

Back in Australia I stuck to the diet rigorously but the constant 'flare-ups' and rapid weight loss (15 kgs in three months) were taking their toll. Just before Christmas 1992 I decided that I could not keep to the therapy any longer. I was at my lowest point. I had given up hope and felt that I would not live to see the end of January 1993. I even contemplated suicide. I did not want my young son to watch me suffer any more.

But God had other plans in mind. He wasn't ready for me, just yet. A friend from Melbourne phoned me and begged me to come and stay with her. She said she wanted to look after me. I gathered what little strength I had and flew to Melbourne on Boxing Day. This was the turning point for me and I owe my friend, Robyn, a very special debt of gratitude. Through her unconditional love and support she very gently picked me up, emotionally and spiritually and put me on my healing path. She introduced me to meditation and Ian Gawler's diet. She encouraged me to attend Ian's 10-day Residential Program. I left there with hope and some courage to fight on.

I attended the 10-day Residential in February 1993 with Cheryl. I found myself surrounded by people who offered me unconditional love and support. Ian taught us to meditate effectively and during those ten days I learnt to take responsibility for my life and my illness.

At this point I would like to state that I believe that I bear at least some responsibility for my cancer. For some time before my diagnosis I was extremely unhappy in my marriage. I had no goals or direction in my life. I spent my life trying to please others. I had even, on a couple of occasions, said to myself, "I bet I get cancer one day!" I made my body an ideal environment for illness.

I came home from The Gawler Foundation with much enthusiasm and a determination that I was going to beat this illness. I had many hurdles to overcome.

My marriage had been very poor before I was diagnosed with cancer. We were on the verge of separating, but once I found out that I had cancer we agreed to try and put aside our problems while I was ill. Ray was very supportive, but we were only 'band-aiding' the problems. We decided to separate in June 1993. I could not work at fixing my marriage while I was working at getting well.

Initially I improved rapidly, but then the stress of having to sell my house and move had a negative effect on me. I began intravenous vitamin C therapy. This helped tremendously. I got back a lot of my energy and was able to lead a fairly normal life.

I returned to The Gawler Foundation every six months to attend the five-day follow-up course. I found these courses extremely helpful. I was able to get back on track with meditation and diet and sort out any other problems I was having. It is easy to lose your way when living a new lifestyle and slip back into old habits, particularly if you are doing it all on your own. I have attended three follow-up courses and honestly believe that they have played an important part in my recovery.

I have had surgery on two more occasions during the past eighteen months. These were for limited removal of lymph nodes in my neck that were becoming a problem. I believe that it is important to use conventional medicine alongside alternative therapies to gain the best possible treatment. Each of us is an individual and we each have to decide which treatment is best for us.

I have had to make many difficult decisions during my healing journey. The most difficult one was deciding to send my eight year old son Paul to live with his father. I found the strain of being a single parent too great. I initially felt a tremendous amount of guilt, but I know that I have made the right decision. I need to put all my energies into getting well. I know that I will miss part of his growing up now, but I know that this will mean that I will be around to see him in years to come.

I have a deep, inner conviction that I will get well. Ian talks about making the transition from 'hope' to 'belief' to 'faith' in our healing journey. I know that I have made that 'leap of faith'. Emotionally and spiritually I feel healed but it may take a while for my physical body to heal.

I am thankful for my cancer. At 33 I was 'shaken by the shoulders' and told to take stock of my life. My illness has been a process of metamorphosis. I have gone from being a woman with no goals and having no direction in my life. My life now has a purpose. I have begun a degree in counselling and I wish to specialise in counselling other people with cancer. We can all learn from each other and so enrich all our healing journeys.

February 1995

Hans Poulsen

Success in the music industry and the sale of my home in Hawthorn in 1972 prompted me to begin a quest that was to last 50 years. Searching for answers to questions like: "What are we doing here?" "What's the world for?" and "Is there some kind of destiny that we are meant to merge with?" were usually incorporated in the lyrics of my songs. Spending three years at the Findhorn community in Scotland, then travelling to America, where I married and my daughter was born.

Suddenly, everything appeared to go haywire. My marriage failed and I wrote this song:

We settled down
a flat in town
and everything was fine.
The band was always round.
I took you so for granted
it never crossed my mind
while I was out saving the world
you might be home crying.
And as you turned away
I heard you say ...
Be easy on the friends who love you
be gentle with the ones who care
Be easy on the friends who love you
be thankful for them while they're there.

The old red Volkswagon slewed around and almost turned over on the snow covered icy wet road in Shutesbury, Massachusetts. The doctors had just told me I had testicular cancer and that I would need an operation straight away.

"When was the moment you knew you were very ill?" (asked Dr Emmett Miller at The Gawler Foundation.) I recalled hanging up the phone to my ex-wife, being denied the access to our daughter that we had agreed on. The pain shot through my joints as I lay back in the chair. I felt totally helpless, confused and drained of the enthusiasm and joy that was my usual state of being. Was I a perfect candidate for cancer?

The operation in itself was a success, but the cancer had already spread into my lungs. Ten tumours on the right side (one the size of a cricket ball) and seven tumours on the left. I was given roughly six months or a few weeks to live, the doctors couldn't tell. It was then something occurred that was to change my life. Rick and Peggy who had put me under their wing suggested I try a therapy session called GIM — or Guided Imagery and Music. A friend of theirs, a Robin Casarjian, who lived in the apartment upstairs had just completed the three years training. I remember the session began with a Beethoven piano concerto. My imagery began to fade with the sheer beauty of Wagner's Loengrin. I could hear Robin turning the tape. The music must have lifted me to a realm we rarely experience.

Rick took me back to the hospital two days later for further X-rays, and the tumours were disappearing before the oncologist's eyes (a Doctor Roger Lang of Mt Aubin Hospital, Boston).

That happened fifteen years ago, almost to the day, and I have been in remission ever since.

Life still had far more to teach me, however, and around 8 p.m. on the 3rd October 1992, I underwent a massive stroke or brain stem haemorrhage in Canada, BC, with a 1% chance of survival. With the perspective that the stroke and subsequent month-long coma have given me, I have written a book with the aid of computers, covering the possible reasons we might get ill and what we might employ for our healing.

Is there an answer? Is there a secret way through life? Illness is certainly a profound teacher. But for us all, while consciousness still exists, there is always the opportunity for more learning with our hearts.

September 1995

Richard Horne

May this privileged sharing of a life's truth without covers or concealment touch others affected by cancer and provide inspiration to anyone who has lost hope or the will to live; lest we forget we are cancer patients and that's OK! My cancer covers nearly 15 years of my life so far — the last year traverses a disposition to suicide through to the path of enlightenment.

This story is dedicated to my darling wife, Valerie, who sat up in a chair at my bedside for four nights following major surgery in 1992 and again in 1994.

Growing up for me in suburban Sydney was mostly unhappy and without much love. To make it worse we were very poor; no car, T.V., record player, telephone or hot running water. Everything I had was second-hand. My self-made billy cart was the best. My father had heart disease from when I was eight and so I took on the gardening, wood chopping, lawn mowing and helping to care for my grandfather who I have been told recently was likely trying to live his cranky life through my body. At 14 I was devastated when my father died. He had become a friend to me by then. I grew angry and bitter, took a part-time job and vowed never to be poor. He left us with nothing. A year later I took a full-time job and went to night school. Nothing was going to stop me becoming a chartered accountant but it was tough — my beautiful five children tell it: "Dad had three jobs at once and a broken axe handle".

Success came — at 30 a partner in a city firm; five years later in one of the big eight — Wow! With 25 years of all this pressure my body's nervous system virtually collapsed. I started transcendental meditation and used the practice just to maintain stability — it seems this was far from enough.

The struggle continued until May 1981. Our then family GP had missed diagnosis until my 12th visit over a six-week period. I had squamous cell carcinoma (S.C.C.) of the floor of the mouth — reasonably rare and without explicable cause! What about 25 years of anxiety, stress and unresolved grief for starters! I knew nothing of cancer (asked hundreds of unanswered questions, like "Why Me?") — nor of other help or support resources. My wife and five children aged 2–14 remained as I did for a long time in shock. My surgeon removed the tumour during six to seven hours of radical surgery with the splitting of my mandible to gain access, hundreds of stitches etc. — yes radical indeed. Afterwards you wonder how you could recover and look reasonably normal. My very dedicated specialist head and neck surgeon admitted he didn't disfigure patients any more than this during surgery — little did either of us know then that worse was to come some years hence.

While I was still in shock from the whole process I went back to work several weeks later. My wife had given up her own social life to care for me. It took a long time to virtually learn to talk again but I got better and was free of cancer for the ensuing 10 years. During that time I worked hard in my own sole accountancy practice and finally built up some wealth from a materialistic based life in many ways, whilst still enjoying my family's growing up. We had a modest holiday beach-house and some great overseas family holidays. In 1986 I intuitively felt the need to change my career, but I was analysis trained so why would I follow my intuitive instincts. Anyway I guess I lacked the courage to make major changes that might involve taking risks. By now it hadn't occurred to me that cancer could return to my life — I'd had my dose — it might happen to someone else but never me.

In 1990 the recession came and with it my worry that a bad property deal and the prospects of my own business and those of my clients failure may lead to a loss of much of my financial treasure. So I again became angry, bitter and resentful, pleading for help in the most arrogant and ridiculous manner. Naturally it wasn't forthcoming and as if I'd wished for it I found in 1991/92 S.C.C. again — this time another primary as before, but a further one in the lower jaw gum. By now surgery techniques included a live transplant of tissue with artery, veins, etc. from my wrist to my mouth, and a skin graft from the thigh to the wrist — another six to seven hour operation; with two surgeons this time (one a micro surgeon). I had learnt little and so again back to work — this time struggling more and with even more resentment and need for help. I made a few changes, but didn't know which way to turn and so continued with angry and resentful attitudes.

The inevitable happened in 1994 again with S.C.C. — this time in the tongue itself and again in the jaw gum. My surgeon told me "I can't operate this time — you won't be up to it and I fear from lack of information from the biopsy that the gum area may be riddled with cancer — go and see the radiotherapist". The radiotherapist thankfully was totally honest: "I can likely cure you of cancer but who'd want to live after I've finished with your treatment". My wife and I sat in the hospital grounds carpark with apparent rationality calculating when and how I could end my life — suicide looked the most practical; maybe euthanasia. Out of this shock state came some exciting prospects. I had some months earlier attended two residential programs at The Gawler Foundation in Melbourne. I had learned about grieving and of forgiveness and had successfully practised these. I had been taught to accept diagnosis not necessarily prognosis, seek information, be responsible for myself, make changes, take risks — we were told why and shown how to do these things and live our own truth not through fabrication and ego and to live a better life even in the face of death.

My mind and memory now began to draw on the incredible experiences I had at The Foundation. Referring back to the copious notes and making contact with Ian Gawler started me on a wonderful campaign. With a newly found G.P. and Ian, hope was restored and choices were emerging. We formulated a program — meditation three hours a day, strict diet observance, herbal concoctions, coffee enemas and a powerhouse of positive thinking. Within six weeks I felt mentally that I might have the cancer beaten, but it still existed physically. I had by then talked through with my surgeon the prospects for surgery. He was generous both with his time and attitude to my changed being.

There was a sense of calm excitement with this surgery that I had now chosen to have and so with volumes of information and hard work, prepared for it. I was to lose the front of my tongue, gum and some jawbone and there were concerns about thereafter both talking and eating. The same two surgeons operated similarly again for six to seven hours — the mandible split, grafts and several more hundreds of stitches. I came out of this surgery with seven tubes penetrating my body — several blood drainage bags, a P.C.A., intravenous drips, a nasal gastro tube and oh yes, a catheter — handy but horrible. From the moment of consciousness this recovery was very, very different. If only I'd known before of what I could do to help myself with pre-op preparations, meditations and positive attitudes.

I had closed my business immediately on diagnosis this time, having learnt the need to create essential time and space to fully address the processes of finding choices, making decisions about my health and my life. This has allowed some clarity and opens opportunities to look at my future — I feel this will be in researching, writing and with cancer patient support.

Epilogue — six months after surgery and now about six months ago, I began a transformation towards enlightenment — I believe this has happened from huge chunks of meditation, being ready to accept change and its associated risks, reading of Buddhist teachings, forceful positive thinking and the willingness to live fully in each moment instead of having my mind, body and soul in different places all the time. I have also learnt to be humble. The result is I now live a life of now and truth without fear of anyone or anything. My fear has been replaced with love.

As I write, external surgery is planned for a week away on a tumour for which biopsies so far are inconclusive. The results will be known soon, but how ordinary they will be — I've learnt to accept the prospect of living with cancer and dying from cancer. Of course much will be done if malignancy shows. Dying, I accept now as not an end but another beginning. I agree with Steve Monegetti's very apt rule "there is a beginning, a middle and another beginning" — thanks Steve.

My love and thanks to my loving and supportive family (whose lives have been greatly affected by my cancers) and to you Ian for your inspiration and great work through The Foundation. I humbly honour my surgeon and present G.P. for their dedication to my needs and the wider common human cause. They have given plenty and given up even more. I hope one day to meet with Pema Chodron, author of *The Wisdom of No Escape* and *Start Where You Are* — for major refocusing on how to let go of 40 years of fear and to live with groundlessness and to the now beautiful journey of the rest of my life no matter what. So be it!

May all sentient beings enjoy with me peace and love.

October 1995

Jill Beardsley

After having been diagnosed with breast cancer and losing all our money in the Pyramid Building Society crash, both happening within 48 hours of each other, my stable secure lifestyle was turned upside-down. Virtually overnight I was left broke and facing death!

My husband Peter and I had just purchased a newsagency, so after my mastectomy I found it necessary to put all considerations about my health on the back burner as we once again strived for financial security.

Two and a half years later when bone secondaries were diagnosed, the full realisation of just how much trouble I was in finally hit home! All the medical profession could offer was life-extending drugs; there certainly wasn't any hope given of ever overcoming the disease. I realised that if I was to get well I would have to find the way myself, and set about finding the people who could help me.

I read Ian Gawler's *You Can Conquer Cancer,* and with great trepidation booked into a Gawler Foundation 10-day residential. What transpired over those ten days was mind boggling. I learned the reason why I had this disease and once I understood that, it was an easy step to realise how I could help myself. I lost my fear of death, I found love, I found peace. I went to the Yarra Valley Living Centre to find out how not to die and came away knowing how to live. Hanging out with Ian for ten days made me realise that he was no mystical, magical guru; he was just your normal, garden variety human being and if he could overcome his disease, then I could overcome mine.

Once home, I threw myself into my new-found life with a passion — diet, meditation, intravenous vitamin C and juices, juices, juices. We hired a full-time assistant for the shop. I rang my friends and told them I wanted no contact with them until I was ready. Every minute of every day was totally committed to and focused on healing. It would be nearly twelve months before I had any real social interaction again. Only then did I feel comfortable enough with my lifestyle and confident that I had my disease under control.

I remained disease free for some eighteen months, during which time I realised two of my life's ambitions. One was learning to scuba dive on the Great Barrier Reef; the other was a family trip to America.

To my horror, a routine bone scan showed that the bone disease was increasing. I thought I had been doing everything right, what more could I possibly do?

About this same time I read Grace Gawler's *Women of Silence*, and then booked in for a five-day Breast Cancer Residential. Grace helped me to realise that although I had made the mind–body connection, I hadn't even touched on the emotional or the spiritual levels.

With Grace's loving encouragement I began to complete my full healing circle.

My disease is once again under control, but I know I still have a long way to go. I have never felt so at ease with myself and with life and believe that so long as I continue with the right blend of Gawler science and medical science, one complementing the other, then I will survive and survive well.

One of the mental imagery exercises I do is to picture myself as I would like to be in my later years. I see myself very clearly as a happy and healthy 101 year old, probably still with blonded hair, dressed in black leathers, and sitting astride a Harley Davidson!

October 1995

Ian & Grace Gawlers' Story

Editor's Note

This history was written for, and published in, The Australian Doctor *to detail the events of my recovery and to clarify what in the past have been misunderstandings regarding these events and their timing. It is written in a fairly matter of fact style! An interview published in the book* Remarkable Recoveries *by Carol Hirschberg and Marc Barash, provides a good balance to this account of what we did. The interview details the care, love and intimacy provided by Grace that were key elements in my healing, elements that partners can generate within themselves and those they care for. The importance of the partner's role, in my case of course Grace's, has often been omitted in articles over the years, with more attention being given to the techniques we used rather than the emotional support generated. Both are necessary to provide the balance and the harmony that is healing!*

In 1975, as a young veterinarian and athlete, aged 24, I had my right leg amputated because of osteogenic sarcoma.

Later that year, inoperable secondaries were confirmed in the right inguinal and mediastinal lymph nodes. In those days, I was told available chemotherapies were of no value and radiotherapy would be palliative at best. The prognosis of 3–6 months was considered reasonable.

I turned to diet and meditation.

Importantly, my wife fully supported my view that cancer could involve a failure of my body's immune system. If we could find a way to reactivate it perhaps I could recover.

We initially followed the Gerson diet. This was exceedingly rigorous and created many problems.

These days, we advise against using the Gerson diet as it is far too demanding in a home setting. However, I do believe it has enough merit to warrant serious study.

I feel sure that nutritional factors helped me a great deal. Many patients report the positive benefits associated with changing their diets. There is a good body of evidence to indicate that nutrition can alter the outcome of cancer. Numerous animal studies confirm the proposition, though studies in humans have been more limited.

I also began meditation with Dr Ainslie Meares. Dr Meares believed that prolonged meditation could reduce cortisol levels, improve immune function and so lead to recovery.

For that first three months my tumours remained static. Then severe sciatic pain forced me to try acupuncture (two treatments only) then palliative radiotherapy (three treatments to my lower lumbar region only). The pain continued to be severe but was then relieved by injections of a mistletoe extract administered by a G.P. interested in natural therapies.

By March 1976, I was suffering severe weight loss (though 1.8m I weighed 54kg), jaundice, night sweats and hydronephrosis of the right kidney (on IVP). The pain was again severe.

At this point my surgeon considered my prognosis to be a couple of weeks.

My wife and I then left for four weeks with faith healers in the Philippines. This was a truly extraordinary experience which challenged all my preconceptions and experience of surgery.

Importantly I came home 6kg heavier, with no pain and feeling I had turned the corner.

In the next six months, while my general health improved, the cancer itself continued to spread and grow. I maintained the modified diet and meditation while my wife did many hours of massage for me. We also investigated many natural therapies.

By late 1976 I had massive secondaries on my sternum, my left lung, lumbar spine; mediastinal and inguinal lymph nodes. Remarkably, I was free of pain and otherwise unaffected by this widespread cancer. However, I reconsidered the medical options.

I was offered experimental chemotherapy based on 'Adriamycin', vincristine and methotrexate. I completed the first round of this protocol in two-and-a-half months but there was little change in my tumour sizes. I then elected to cease treatment despite warnings of a rapid rebound.

We returned to the Philippines for three months, travelling then to India. In May 1977, the holy man Sai Baba told me: "You are already cured, don't worry."

This was another major turning point, as it helped me to dispel doubts and be fully confident of recovery.

I had no more medical treatment but continued, fully committed, to the self-help regimen as described.

By June 1978 all visible lesions had subsided. Tests in Adelaide confirmed that there was no evidence of active cancer, but I did have TB. I responded rapidly to standard TB treatment, and my case was reported by Dr Meares.

Grace and I moved to Yarra Junction, Victoria in 1980. We have had four children since chemotherapy.

Obviously this is a complex history. I am often asked what cured me, and I reply that it was a combined result.

I have no doubt that the medical treatment on its own would have been unsuccessful. My recovery demanded a great deal of effort from both myself and my wife.

In 1981, my wife and I began an innovative cancer support group based on our experiences. At that time little was being offered to people affected by cancer who wanted to help themselves. Patients were being left to fend for themselves. Hope was often denied and the myth of cancer as a death sentence prevailed.

We were keen to redress these painful problems and felt we had something important to offer. The main ingredients of our approach were (and still are) good nutrition, developing a positive state of mind, meditation and mutual support.

Our patient-based programs gained wide interest.

In 1983 we founded the non-profit, non-denominational charitable organisation The Gawler Foundation to extend this work and left our veterinary practice.

In 1984 I detailed our approach in *You Can Conquer Cancer.* The book was launched by Sir Edward 'Weary' Dunlop who remained a strong supporter of our work.

In the same year, being keen on scientific evaluation, I unsuccessfully approached the Peter MacCallum Cancer Institute in Melbourne and the Victorian Anti-Cancer Council for help with research. Like many self-help groups, our resources were limited and we could get no outside assistance at that time.

In 1987, we began developing our own extensive in-house database with a view to follow-up research. In the same year I was awarded the Order of Australia medal for services to the community and published a detailed account of our meditation and positive thinking methods in *Peace of Mind.*

The Gawler Foundation

Two Types of Programs

Based upon the Gawlers' story and developed by the experience and knowledge gained over the years, The Gawler Foundation is able to offer a wide range of programs with a dual emphasis. Direct, practical assistance is provided for people affected by cancer. As a logical extension of this work, direction is also given to those interested in prevention and total health — for body, mind and spirit.

The Gawler Foundation is a non-profit, non-denominational Incorporated Association registered in Victoria since 1983. It is a charity managed by a voluntary committee. All donations are tax deductible.

Since 1983, over 10,000 people have attended The Gawler Foundation's programs. Currently Grace is working independently from, but in co-operation with The Foundation. She has recently founded "Ellimatta" Women's Wholistic Health Care and is in private consulting practice, conducting residential programs for women with breast cancer and national and International seminars.

The Yarra Valley Living Centre

Located one hour east of Melbourne, amidst the peace and tranquility of the Yarra Valley, The Gawler Foundation's headquarters, named the Yarra Valley Living Centre, is truly a healing centre with a difference. Here people learn far more than what can be done for them, they learn what they can do for themselves! How to help themselves and support each other. How to work in effective partnership with their health professionals. How to find peace of mind, personal contentment and fulfilment. Indeed, this is a very special place for life.

A New Approach to Cancer that Offers Real Hope!

The Gawler Foundation's support system is integrated and complete. Experience shows that many people, like those included in this book have been able to use their own resources effectively to overcome the many challenges of cancer. The Foundation's programs offer patients, their families and friends the opportunity to learn how — in a loving and caring environment, supported by dedicated staff.

In any situation there will be people who will cope in an average way, others do poorly, some do exceptionally well. Until recently, it was left to chance as to how well people affected by cancer managed. The Gawler Foundation's work has changed that. There is now a program that teaches cancer patients, their families and friends how to be exceptionally effective — and supports them in their efforts.

What are the Hallmarks of Success?

Those who have experienced these wonderful results have:

- Made an intensive and prolonged personal effort;
- Enjoyed vital, healthy lifestyle changes;
- Received effective support from family, groups and individual counsellors;
- Learnt how to get the best results from appropriate medical treatment.

As a group they have come to demonstrate:

- A quiet but powerful positive self esteem.
- A sense of purpose and meaning in their life.
- Effective personal discipline in applying self-help techniques.
- A personally satisfying, sustained sense of peace of mind.

What To Do Next

More detailed information and brochures are available from The Gawler Foundation. Ian's books *You Can Conquer Cancer* and *Peace of Mind* and Grace's *Women of Silence* are an excellent starting point. Tapes are available also and can be very helpful. You might like to request a specific information package. We recommend everyone to take advantage of our programs as soon as possible after diagnosis. Wherever possible patients are advised to attend with a support person.

YOU CAN CONQUER CANCER

If you think we can help you — reach out and get in touch.
Call us Monday – Friday, 9 a.m. to 5 p.m.,
Talk with us, perhaps visit the bookshop, find out how we can help.

LOCATION:

The Yarra Valley Living Centre,
Rayner Court, Yarra Junction,
Victoria 3797 Australia.
Telephone **(059) 67 1730** Fax: **(059) 67 1715**

Further Reading

Further reading about remarkable recoveries and inspiring healing of cancer:

You Can Conquer Cancer, Ian Gawler, Hill of Content, 1984

Peace of Mind, Ian Gawler, Hill of Content, 1987

Women of Silence, The Emotional Healing of Breast Cancer, Grace Gawler, Hill of Content, 1994

Spontaneous Remission, An annotated bibliography, Brendan O'Regan & Caryle Hirschberg, Institute of Noetic Sciences, 1993

Remarkable Recovery, What Extraordinary Healings Tell us About Getting Well and Staying Well, by Caryle Hirschberg and Marc Barasch, Hodder Headline, 1995

Where There's Hope, Patricia Gilishenen, 1990

The Healing Path, A Soul Approach to Illness, Marc Barasch, Penguin, 1993

Flowers in Winter, Defeating Cancer, A Westerner's Chinese Journey, Sir William Keyes, Allen & Unwin, 1995

Anatomy of an Illness, Norman Cousins, Bantam, 1979

Cancer as a Turning Point, Lawrence LeShan, Penguin, 1994

Why Me, Garrett Porter & Patricia Norris, Stillpoint Publishing, 1985

My Triumph Over Cancer, Beata Bishop, Keats, 1986

Love, Medicine and Miracles, Bernie Siegel, Arrow, 1986.